ESSENTIAL

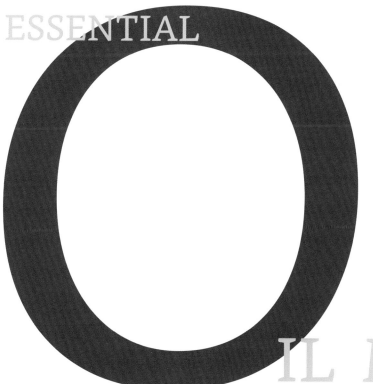

IL MAGIC

2nd Edition

Essential Oil Magic
Easy-to-Use Guidebook + Tearaway Protocols

v2.0 Edition October 2018

ISBN: 978-0-9993689-3-0

Published by:

Oil Magic Publishing
Cheyenne, Wyoming
contact@oilmagicbook.com

Disclaimer to Readers:

This book is for reference purposes only. The information contained has not been evaluated by the US Food and Drug Administration, or by other government entities. It is not provided to diagnose, treat, cure, or prevent any disease, illness, or any injured condition of the body.

The authors and publisher of this book are not liable for any misconception or misuse of the information provided. They are not responsible or liable for any person or entity in regards to any damage, loss, or injury caused, or supposed to be caused, either directly or indirectly from the use of the contents of this book.

This book is not intended to be a substitute for medical counseling. Anyone suffering from any illness, injury, or disease should consult a qualified healthcare professional.

About this book

This book is for the lovers of doing things naturally. You can create magic when you have the right ingredients, and essential oils seem almost just like that: magical.

Use this guide as your first go-to. Turn to nature as your first resort, and remember that you also have the power of western medicine when needed.

When you make a habit of using natural remedies like essential oils, you learn that you have the ability to create the wellness you want. Your oils are a treasure trove. They're versatile, they rarely produce side-effects, and they're friendly to your pocket book when you compare them to doctor visits and medication costs.

Enjoy all the things your oils can do for you. Enjoy the aromas, and have fun blending oils to make your own aromas. Try creative DIY projects, or even put a drop of oil in your cooking or baking.

Most importantly, see what happens to your confidence as you learn to trust nature and yourself with your family's wellness.

Use the Ailments section as a quick reference guide to find natural remedies for your health concerns. Discover the top uses of popular essential oils in the Single Oils and Oil Blends sections. Use the Protocols section to get serious results. And share the tearaway protocols in Protocols for Sharing with friends!

Have fun creating your magic.

Table of *Contents*

Essential & *Advanced*

This book you hold in your hands is the perfect starter reference guide for essential oils. It contains the most essential knowledge to use essential oils and supplements to tackle common health challenges.

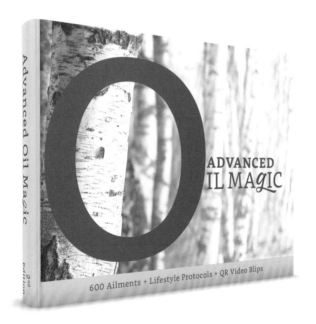

ADVANCED Oil Magic is the comprehensive companion to Essential Oil Magic. Just as easy to use; tons more valuable information.

www.oilmagicbook.com

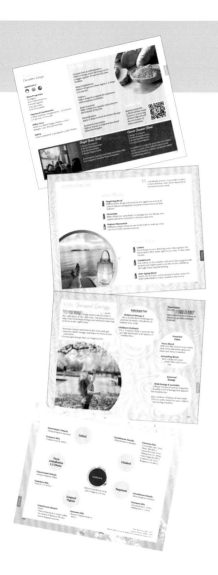

> 600 quick reference Ailments & Conditions

> Uses & oil hacks for even more Single Oils & Oil Blends

> Hundreds of recipes, diffuser blends, & DIY's

> Lifestyle Protocols

> 105 serious Ailment Protocols

> Incredible Emotions & Energy usage

> Gorgeous Essential Oil Science made useful & practical

> QR Video Blips on your favorite essential oils

Section 1

Simplified
Usage Guide

Uses

1 Aromatic

Diffuse
Put 4-8 drops in a diffuser to spread the oil throughout the room.

From Hands
Inhale a couple drops from cupped hands.

From Bottle
Enjoy the aroma directly from the bottle.

2 Topical

Neat
Apply certain oils directly to skin without dilution.

Dilute
Dilute with Fractionated Coconut Oil or other carrier oil/lotion as needed.

Roller Bottle
Put 10-20 drops in a roller bottle. Fill the rest with Fractionated Coconut Oil.

3 Internal

Veggie Capsule
Put oils in an empty veggie cap, and take with water.

Drink with Water
Drink 1-2 drops with water (for oils with a friendly taste).

Most brands of oils are not safe for internal use. Be sure yours has undergone strict gas chromatography and mass spectrometry to ensure purity and chemical soundness.

Safety

Children

Essential oils are safe to use with children in smaller amounts. The smaller the child, the less essential oil needed. Use this chart as a general guideline for use with children.

Age	Topical Dilution Ratio*	Internal Use
Birth - 12 months	1:30	1 drop (3-12 drops in 12 hours)
1-5 years	1:20	1 drop (3-12 drops in 12 hours)
6-11 years	1:15	1-2 drops (3-12 drops in 12 hours)

*essential oil : carrier oil

Medication

Always consult with a physician if you have questions about using an essential oil with a medication. While certain foods may interact with medications, essential oils frequently require less restraint because of the chemical makeup of the oil vs. the food.

Pregnancy

Essential oils are wonderful for pregnancy support. Oils can be used in smaller doses, and certain oils should be avoided: Birch[ATI], Cassia[TI], Cinnamon[TI], Cypress[I], Eucalyptus[I], Rosemary[ATI], Thyme[ATI], Wintergreen[TI].

Sensitive Skin

Dilute as needed for sensitive skin. Apply to the bottoms of feet to avoid sensitivity.

Preference & Purpose

Remember that while essential oils have a most useful purpose, you should also enjoy what you use! Enjoying the use of oils makes it easier to create lifestyle habits with them.

If you love the smell of an essential oil, use away! If you don't love the smell, try an application method that limits exposure to the fragrance (like in a veggie cap or on the bottoms of feet), or look for a different oil that has similar properties.

Blending

Remember that you can't break your oils. If you experiment with blending, but don't succeed, try again. You'll learn the smells that resonate best with you.

Sometimes you'll find yourself in need of an oil you may not love. Try combining it with another oil to create a fragrance you enjoy.

Here are some blending tips:

- Pay attention to low, mid, and high notes in your oils for a well-rounded fragrance. (e.g. Vetiver is a low note, Lavender is a mid note, and Lemon is a high note.)

- Add FCO to your blends to help the fragrance last longer.

- When layering oils topically (using multiple oils one on top of the other), the oils on top will generally smell the strongest.

How much oil should I use?

Discover what works best for your body. Take heed of the safety warnings for each oil in this book. *Remember - small amounts more frequently tend to produce the best results.*

Section 2

Ailments & Conditions

Acid Reflux

Take 2-4 drops internally or rub over stomach as needed.

Peppermint [T I]
Digestive Blend [T I]
Ginger [T I]
Cardamom [T I]
Digestion Tablets [I]
Protocol on pg. 172

Acne/Blemishes

Apply a drop topically to affected areas 1-2x daily. Add 2-3 drops to facial lotion and apply after cleansing routine.

Melaleuca [T]
Skin Clearing Blend [T]
Juniper Berry [T]
Neroli [T]
Lavender [T]
Protocol on pg. 160

ADD/ADHD

Apply a few drops on forehead and back of neck; inhale a few drops from cupped hands.

Focus Blend [A T]
Vetiver [A T I]
Reassuring Blend [A T I]
Frankincense [A T I]
Grounding Blend [A T]
Protocol on pg. 161

Adrenal Fatigue

Massage 1-3 drops onto lower back over adrenals, or inhale from cupped hands. Take 1-3 drops internally as needed.

Basil [A T I]
Juniper Berry [A T I]
Rosemary [A T I]
Geranium [A T I]
Ylang Ylang [A T I]
Protocol on pg. 161

Aging

Apply 1-3 drops to target areas. Combine 2-8 drops with facial lotion or carrier oil and apply after cleansing.

Anti-Aging Blend [T]
Frankincense [T]
Cedarwood [T]
Sandalwood [T]
Vitality Trio [I]

Alertness

Apply 1-2 drops to forehead, temples, or base of skull as needed; inhale a few drops from cupped hands.

Peppermint [A T I]
Frankincense [A T I]
Basil [A T I]
Rosemary [A T I]
Focus Blend [A T]

Allergies (Seasonal, Pet Dander)

Apply to back of neck, on bridge of nose, or chest as needed; use a drop under the tongue; diffuse several drops.

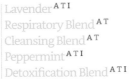

Lavender [A T I]
Respiratory Blend [A T]
Cleansing Blend [A T]
Peppermint [A T I]
Detoxification Blend [A T I]
Protocol on pg. 162

Alzheimer's/ Dementia

Massage 1-2 drops into scalp daily; ingest 2-4 drops 1-2x daily; supplement daily.

Frankincense [A T I]
Rosemary [A T I]
Cellular Complex [A T I]
Rose [A T]
Vitality Trio [T]
Protocol on pg. 163

Anemia

Apply 1-3 drops to bottoms of feet and inside of wrists; take a few drops internally; inhale from cupped hands periodically.

Protective Blend ᴬ ᵀ ᴵ
Basil ᴬ ᵀ ᴵ
Lemon ᴬ ᵀ ᴵ
Lavender ᴬ ᵀ ᴵ
Vitality Trio ᵀ

Anger

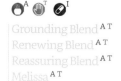

Apply 1-3 drops to temples and chest; inhale a few drops from cupped hands as needed.

Grounding Blend ᴬ ᵀ
Renewing Blend ᴬ ᵀ
Reassuring Blend ᴬ ᵀ
Melissa ᴬ ᵀ
Magnolia ᴬ ᵀ

Ankle Swelling

Massage ankles with 2-4 drops diluted with carrier oil if desired.

Juniper Berry ᵀ
Grapefruit ᵀ
Lemongrass ᵀ
Soothing Blend ᵀ
Tension Blend ᵀ

Anorexia

Apply 1-3 drops to stomach area or inhale from cupped hands as needed.

Grapefruit ᴬ ᵀ
Ginger ᴬ ᵀ
Invigorating Blend ᴬ ᵀ
Joyful Blend ᴬ ᵀ
Uplifting Blend ᴬ ᵀ

Anxiety

Apply 1-3 drops to bottoms of feet, chest, or temples, or inhale from cupped hands as needed; use a drop under the tongue.

Grounding Blend ᴬ ᵀ
Vetiver ᴬ ᵀ ᴵ
Reassuring Blend ᴬ ᵀ
Bergamot ᴬ ᵀ ᴵ
Frankincense ᴬ ᵀ ᴵ
Protocol on pg. 163

Apathy

Apply 1-3 drops to bottoms of feet, chest, or temples, or inhale from cupped hands as needed. Also diffuse several drops.

Patchouli ᴬ ᵀ
Neroli ᴬ ᵀ
Peppermint ᴬ ᵀ
Ylang Ylang ᴬ ᵀ
Renewing Blend ᴬ ᵀ

Appetite Suppressant

Apply 1-3 drops to stomach, chest, bottoms of feet, or inside of wrists or take 2-4 drops internally.

Metabolic blend ᴬ ᵀ ᴵ
Peppermint ᴬ ᵀ ᴵ
Grapefruit ᴬ ᵀ ᴵ
Ginger ᴬ ᵀ ᴵ
Wild Orange ᴬ ᵀ ᴵ

Arthritic Pain

Apply 1-3 drops and massage into affected areas with lotion or carrier oil as needed.

Soothing Blend ᵀ
Copaiba ᵀ
Wintergreen ᵀ
Massage Blend ᵀ
Cellular Complex ᵀ
Protocol on pg. 163

15

Asthma

Apply 1-3 drops topically to chest, neck, under nose, and on bridge of nose, or inhale from cupped hands as needed.

Respiratory Blend [A T]
Eucalyptus [A T]
Peppermint [A T]
Roman Chamomile [A T]
Lavender [A T]
Protocol on pg. 164

Athlete's Foot

Apply 1-3 drops to area between toes and around toenails 2-3x daily. Ingest 1-3 drops of melaleuca or oregano once a day (no more than 10 days).

Melaleuca [T I]
Oregano [T I]
Skin Clearing Blend [T]
Geranium [T I]
Lemon [T I]

Autism/Asperger's

Apply 1-3 drops to bottoms of feet and back of neck. Ingest 1-3 drops of Cilantro or Cellular Complex 1-2x daily.

Frankincense [A T I]
Focus Blend [A T]
Cilantro [A T I]
Rose [A T]
Cellular Complex [A T I]
Protocol on pg. 164

Autoimmune Disorders

Apply 1-3 drops to stomach, chest, bottoms of feet, or inside of wrists. Ingest 2-4 drops 3x daily.

Cellular Complex [T I]
Detoxification Blend [T I]
Frankincense [T I]
Anti-Aging Blend [T]
Vitality Trio [I]

Autointoxication

Apply 1-3 drops to stomach, chest, bottoms of feet, or inside of wrists. Ingest 1-3 drops 2-3x daily for additional support.

Detoxification Blend [A T I]
Cilantro [A T I]
Thyme [A T I]
Grapefruit [A T I]
Geranium [A T I]

Back Pain

Apply 1-3 drops and massage into affected areas as needed. Use a carrier oil or lotion for increased efficacy. Take 2 capsules of Cellular Complex 2-3x daily.

Soothing Blend [A T]
Massage Blend [A T]
Turmeric [A T I]
Copaiba [A T I]
Polyphenol Complex [I]
Protocol on pg. 164

Bacterial Infection

Apply 1-3 drops with a carrier oil to affected areas as needed. Ingest 1-3 drops every 2-3 hours for systemic/internal infections.

Oregano [A T I]
Thyme [A T I]
Protective Blend [A T I]
Melaleuca [A T I]
Pink Pepper [A T I]

Balance Problems

Apply 1-3 drops topically to forehead, temples, back of neck, and behind the ears or inhale from cupped hands. Ingest 1-3 drops of Ginger as needed.

Grounding Blend [A T]
Peppermint [A T I]
Ginger [A T I]
Basil [A T I]
Cypress [A T]

Bed-wetting

Massage 2-4 drops over bladder and kidneys before bedtime.

Cypress [T]
Black Pepper [T]
Ylang Ylang [T]
Lemongrass [T]
Roman Chamomile [T]

Bee Sting

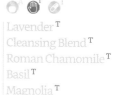

Apply 1-2 drops topically to sting or bite several times daily until symptoms cease.

Lavender [T]
Cleansing Blend [T]
Roman Chamomile [T]
Basil [T]
Magnolia [T]

Bell's Palsy

Ingest 2-4 drops every 2-3 hours as needed; apply 1-3 drops topically.

Clove [T I]
Melissa [T I]
Frankincense [T I]
Thyme [T I]
Vitality Trio [I]

Bipolar Disorder

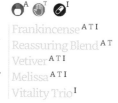

Apply 1-3 drops to bottoms of feet, chest, or temples, or inhale from cupped hands as needed.

Frankincense [A T I]
Reassuring Blend [A T]
Vetiver [A T I]
Melissa [A T I]
Vitality Trio [I]
Protocol on pg. 165

Bladder Control

Apply 1-3 drops topically over bladder and kidneys as needed. Add 1-2 drops to drinking water and sip throughout the day.

Rosemary [T I]
Juniper Berry [T I]
Cypress [T]
Marjoram [T I]
Sandalwood [T I]

Bleeding

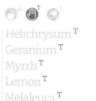

Apply a drop topically to affected area as needed.

Helichrysum [T]
Geranium [T]
Myrrh [T]
Lemon [T]
Melaleuca [T]

Blisters on Feet

Apply a few drops topically to affected area.

Lavender [T]
Frankincense [T]
Patchouli [T]
Melaleuca [T]
Myrrh [T]

Bloating

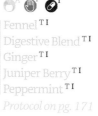

Apply 1-3 drops to stomach, rubbing in a clockwise direction. Use 1-3 drops internally as needed.

Fennel [T I]
Digestive Blend [T I]
Ginger [T I]
Juniper Berry [T I]
Peppermint [T I]
Protocol on pg. 171

Blood Clotting

Apply 1-3 drops to affected area or ingest a few drops internally as needed.

Wintergreen ᵀ ᴵ
Helichrysum ᵀ ᴵ
Birch ᵀ ᴵ
Peppermint ᵀ ᴵ
Ginger ᵀ ᴵ

Blood Pressure (high)

Apply 2-4 drops to stomach, chest, bottoms of feet, or inside of wrists; ingest 2-4 drops 2x daily.

Cypress ᴬ ᵀ
Marjoram ᴬ ᵀ ᴵ
Lemon ᴬ ᵀ ᴵ
Ylang Ylang ᴬ ᵀ ᴵ
Jasmine ᴬ ᵀ
Protocol on pg. 165

Blood Pressure (low)

Apply 1-3 drops to stomach, chest, bottoms of feet, or inside of wrists, or ingest a few drops as needed.

Helichrysum ᴬ ᵀ ᴵ
Frankincense ᴬ ᵀ ᴵ
Jasmine ᴬ ᵀ
Cedarwood ᴬ ᵀ
Vitality Trio ᴵ

Blood Sugar (low)

Apply 1-3 drops to stomach, chest, bottoms of feet, or inside of wrists, or ingest 1-3 drops as needed.

Cinnamon ᵀ ᴵ
Melissa ᵀ ᴵ
Cassia ᵀ ᴵ
Wild Orange ᵀ ᴵ
Vitality Trio ᴵ

Blurred Vision

Mix oils in a roller bottle with carrier oil and carefully apply around eyes 2-4x daily.

Clary Sage ᵀ
Helichrysum ᵀ
Anti-Aging Blend ᵀ
Cellular Complex ᵀ
Lavender ᵀ

Body Odor

Take 3-5 drops of Cilantro, Detoxification Blend, or Dill at least once daily. Apply 1-3 drops on bottoms of feet.

Cilantro ᵀ ᴵ
Detoxification Blend ᵀ ᴵ
Dill ᵀ ᴵ
Melaleuca ᵀ ᴵ
Petitgrain ᵀ ᴵ
Protocol on pg. 169

Boils

Apply 1-3 drops topically to affected areas several times daily.

Melaleuca ᵀ
Skin Clearing Blend ᵀ
Lavender ᵀ
Myrrh ᵀ
Bergamot ᵀ

Bone Pain/Break

Apply 3-5 drops topically to affected areas as needed. Massage with lotion or carrier oil to improve efficacy.

Soothing Blend ᵀ
Wintergreen ᵀ
Birch ᵀ
Helichrysum ᵀ
Bone Nutrient Complex ᴵ

Ailments

Brain Fog

Apply 1-3 drops to forehead, temples, back of neck, and behind ears or inhale from cupped hands as needed.

Peppermint [A T I]
Frankincense [A T I]
Lemon [A T I]
Rosemary [A T I]
Vitality Trio [I]

Brain Injury

Apply a few drops topically to forehead, temples, base of skull, and behind the ears or diffuse into the air and inhale. Take a few drops internally as needed.

Frankincense [A T I]
Cellular Complex [A T I]
Grounding Blend [A T]
Sandalwood [A T I]
Vitality Trio [I]

Ailments

Breastfeeding
(increase milk)

Massage 1-3 drops with carrier oil over breasts and apply to bottoms of feet or take internally when needed.

Fennel [T I]
Clary Sage [T I]
Basil [T I]
Vitality Trio [I]
Bone Nutrient Complex [I]
Protocol on pg. 168

Brittle Nails

Apply 1-2 drops to nail bed once daily. Use supplements consistently for long-term benefits.

Lemon [T]
Helichrysum [T]
Frankincense [T]
Bone Nutrient Complex [I]
Vitality Trio [I]

Bronchitis

Apply 2-4 drops to chest and neck area, gargle hourly, or inhale from cupped hands as needed.

Respiratory Blend [A T]
Cardamom [A T I]
Lime [A T I]
Roman Chamomile [A T I]
Eucalyptus [A T]
Protocol on pg. 157

Bruising

Apply 2-4 drops to bruise area. Use carrier oil if desired. Reapply 2-4x daily.

Tension Blend [T]
Soothing Blend [T]
Helichrysum [T]
Cypress [T]
Anti-Aging Blend [T]

Bunions

Apply 2-4 drops with carrier oil to affected area or joint as needed.

Lemon [T]
Soothing Blend [T]
Copaiba [T]
Peppermint [T]
Cypress [T]

Burns

Apply 2-4 drops to affected area hourly or as needed. For more severe, mix 2-8 drops with 4 oz witch hazel and apply as needed.

Lavender [T]
Frankincense [T]
Helichrysum [T]
Anti-Aging Blend [T]
Cedarwood [T]

Cancer

Ingest 3-5 drops 3-5x daily. Apply topically if appropriate. Diffuse several drops. Supplement for added support.

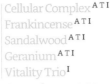

Cellular Complex [A T I]
Frankincense [A T I]
Sandalwood [A T I]
Geranium [A T I]
Vitality Trio [I]
Protocol on pg. 166

Candida

Apply 2-4 drops over abdomen and bottoms of feet. Take 3-5 drops in a capsule at least twice daily until symptoms subside.

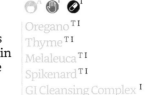

Oregano [T I]
Thyme [T I]
Melaleuca [T I]
Spikenard [T I]
GI Cleansing Complex [I]
Protocol on pg. 166

Canker Sores

Apply a drop diluted with carrier oil directly to canker sore or gargle several times daily until sore is gone.

Melaleuca [T I]
Protective Blend [T I]
Oregano [T I]
Melissa [T I]
Frankincense [T I]
Protocol on pg. 166

Cardiovascular Disease

Apply 2-4 drops over chest 3x daily. Ingest 3-5 drops as needed.

Cellular Complex [T I]
Geranium [T I]
Black Pepper [T I]
Coriander [T I]
Cypress [T]

Carpal Tunnel

Apply 2-4 drops to affected area several times daily. Massage with carrier oil or lotion for improved efficacy.

Soothing Blend [T]
Wintergreen [T]
Lemongrass [T]
Marjoram [T]
Oregano [T]

Cartilage Injury

Apply 1-3 drops to affected area several times daily. Massage with carrier oil or lotion for improved efficacy.

Soothing Blend [T]
Lemongrass [T]
Frankincense [T]
Helichrysum [T]
Copaiba [T]

Cavities

Apply 1-2 drops directly on tooth 2x daily. Dilute with carrier oil if necessary.

Clove [T I]
Protective Blend [T I]
Melaleuca [T I]
Bone Nutrient Complex [I]
Vitality Trio [I]

Cellulite (Fat Deposits)

Massage 4-8 drops onto target areas daily, especially before exercising. Add to drinking water and consume throughout the day.

Metabolic Blend [T I]
Grapefruit [T I]
Lemon [T I]
Juniper Berry [T I]
Cinnamon [T I]
Protocol on pg. 181

Ailments

Chapped Skin

Apply a drop or two to affected area as often as needed. Use a carrier oil to increase efficacy.

Myrrh [T]
Roman Chamomile [T]
Anti-Aging Blend [T]
Cedarwood [T]
Magnolia [T]

Charley Horse

Massage 1-3 drops onto area of concern. Use a carrier oil or lotion for improved efficacy.

Massage Blend [T]
Soothing Blend [T]
Marjoram [T]
Black Pepper [T]
Bergamot [T]

Ailments

Chest Pain

Apply 1-3 drops topically to chest or ingest at least twice daily.

Cellular Complex [T I]
Protective Blend [T I]
Lemon [T I]
Wild Orange [T I]
Marjoram [T I]

Chicken Pox

Dilute 2-4 drops with a carrier oil and dab lightly on spots a couple times a day or ingest for immune support.

Lavender [T I]
Thyme [T I]
Melaleuca [T I]
Cellular Complex [T I]
Melissa [T I]

Chiggers

Dilute 2-4 drops with a carrier oil and dab lightly on bites a couple times a day.

Outdoor Blend [T]
Lemongrass [T]
Melaleuca [T]
Detoxification Blend [T]
Arborvitae [T]

Cholesterol (high)

Apply 2-4 drops to chest area, bottoms of feet, or inside of wrists; ingest 2-4 drops once daily.

Cellular Complex [T I]
Lemon [T I]
Rosemary [T I]
Detoxification Blend [T I]
Vitality Trio [I]
Protocol on pg. 167

Chronic Fatigue

Apply 2-4 drops to chest area, bottoms of feet, or inside of wrists; inhale 1-3 drops from cupped hands; supplement regularly for long-term benefits.

Lemon [A T I]
Melissa [A T I]
Basil [A T I]
Energy & Stamina Complex [I]
Vitality Trio [I]
Protocol on pg. 171

Chronic Pain

Apply 1-3 drops to affected areas as needed, using carrier oil for improved efficacy; supplement regularly for long-term care.

Soothing Blend [A T]
Copaiba [A T I]
Cellular Complex [A T I]
Turmeric [A T I]
Vitality Trio [I]

Circulation (poor)

Apply 1-3 drops to bottoms of feet; ingest 1-3 drops twice daily or as needed.

Cypress [T I]
Ginger [T I]
Black Pepper [T I]
Cellular Complex [T I]
Energy & Stamina Complex [I]

Cold Extremities

Apply 2-4 drops to bottoms of feet, chest area, and inside of wrists; ingest 2-4 drops daily as needed.

Cypress [A T I]
Black Pepper [A T I]
Cinnamon [A T I]
Protective Blend [A T I]
Energy & Stamina Complex [I]

Colic

Dilute 1-2 drops with a carrier oil and apply topically to stomach and back before baby goes to sleep.

Digestive Blend [T]
Peppermint [T]
Fennel [T]
Neroli [T]
Roman Chamomile [T]

Congestion

Apply 1-3 drops to back of neck, under nose, on bridge of nose, or chest; inhale 1-3 drops from cupped hands as needed. Also gargle a drop.

Respiratory Blend [A T]
Lemon [A T I]
Rosemary [A T I]
Cardamom [A T I]
Lime [A T I]

Cold (common)

Ingest 3-5 drops 3-4x daily until symptoms subside. Diffuse several drops. Supplement regularly for long-term benefits.

Protective Blend [A T I]
Respiratory Blend [A T]
Oregano [A T I]
Melissa [A T I]
Thyme [A T I]
Protocol on pg. 168

Cold Sores

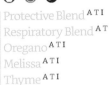

Dilute with carrier oil and apply a drop to affected area as needed.

Melissa [T]
Protective Blend [T]
Melaleuca [T]
Clove [T]
Frankincense [T]
Protocol on pg. 168

Concussion

Apply 2-4 drops to forehead, temples, base of skull, and behind the ears; inhale 1-3 drops from cupped hands; take 2-5 drops internally for a few days.

Frankincense [A T I]
Bergamot [A T I]
Cypress [A T]
Copaiba [A T I]
Rosemary [A T I]

Constipation

Massage 2-4 drops over abdomen, moving in a clockwise fashion. Repeat as desired every 5-10 minutes as needed. Ingest 2-4 drops for additional support.

Digestive Blend [T I]
Ginger [T I]
Marjoram [T I]
Cilantro [T I]
Fennel [T I]
Protocol on pg. 171

Cortisol (heightened)

Apply 1-3 drops to back of neck, under nose, on bridge of nose, or chest as needed; ingest 2-4 drops; inhale from cupped hands.

Lavender ^{A T I}
Basil ^{A T I}
Bergamot ^{A T I}
Marjoram ^{A T I}
Neroli ^{A T}

Protocol on pg. 179

Cough

Apply 1-3 drops to chest, back of neck, under nose, or on bridge of nose, as needed; inhale from cupped hands; gargle a drop.

Respiratory Blend ^{A T}
Rosemary ^{A T I}
Peppermint ^{A T I}
Lemon ^{A T I}
Cardamom ^{A T I}

Protocol on pg. 168

Cramps

Massage 2-4 drops into affected areas as needed. Use with carrier oil to improve efficacy.

Soothing Blend ^T
Massage Blend ^T
Arborvitae ^T
Women's Monthly Blend ^T
Peppermint ^T

Croup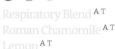

Dilute with carrier oil and apply 1-3 drops to baby's chest and back as needed. Diffuse several drops.

Respiratory Blend ^{A T}
Roman Chamomile ^{A T}
Lemon ^{A T}
Sandalwood ^{A T}
Wild Orange ^{A T}

Crying

Apply 1-2 drops to front of shirt or sleeve, or diffuse several drops.

Lavender ^{A T}
Wild Orange ^{A T}
Reassuring Blend ^{A T}
Roman Chamomile ^{A T}
Restful Blend ^{A T}

Cuts

Dilute 1-2 drops with a carrier oil and apply to affected area a couple times daily.

Melaleuca ^T
Lavender ^T
Helichrysum ^T
Myrrh ^T
Cedarwood ^T

Cystic Fibrosis

Apply 1-3 drops to chest and under nose; inhale from cupped hands as needed.

Frankincense ^{A T}
Respiratory Blend ^{A T}
Arborvitae ^{A T}
Eucalyptus ^{A T}
Melaleuca ^{A T}

Cysts

Apply 2-4 drops to affected area 3x daily or as needed.

Oregano ^T
Frankincense ^T
Thyme ^T
Tangerine ^T
Cellular Complex ^T

Dandruff

Dilute 2-6 drops in carrier oil and massage into scalp. Rinse after 60 minutes.

Melaleuca ^T
Cedarwood ^T
Rosemary ^T
Myrrh ^T
Petitgrain ^T

Dehydrated Skin

Apply 2-4 drops with carrier oil to affected area as needed. Use with lotion for improved efficacy.

Cedarwood ^T
Captivating Blend ^T
Myrrh ^T
Sandalwood ^T
Anti-Aging Blend ^T

Dementia

Apply 2-4 drops to forehead, temples, base of skull, and behind the ears; take internally as needed; inhale from cupped hands as needed.

Frankincense ^{A T I}
Cellular Complex ^{A T I}
Rose ^{A T I}
Rosemary ^{A T I}
Peppermint ^{A T I}
Protocol on pg. 163

Depression

Apply 2-4 drops to forehead and temples; place a drop of Frankincense on thumb and press to roof of mouth; inhale from cupped hands as needed.

Joyful Blend ^{A T}
Frankincense ^{A T I}
Uplifting Blend ^{A T}
Melissa ^{A T I}
Vitality Trio ^I
Protocol on pg. 169

Detoxification

Apply 3-5 drops to bottoms of feet and inside of wrists; ingest 2-4 drops a few times daily; supplement regularly for improved cleansing.

Detoxification Blend ^{T I}
Cilantro ^{T I}
Lemon ^{T I}
Grapefruit ^{T I}
Detox Herbal Complex ^I
Protocol on pg. 170

Diabetes

Apply a couple drops over pancreas and bottoms of feet daily; take a few drops internally.

Protective Blend ^{T I}
Metabolic Blend ^{T I}
Cinnamon ^{T I}
Coriander ^{T I}
Ginger ^{T I}
Protocol on pg. 170

Diaper Rash

Dilute 1-3 drops with carrier oil and apply to affected area several times daily until rash disappears.

Lavender ^T
Roman Chamomile ^T
Ylang Ylang ^T
Coriander ^T
Cedarwood ^T

Diarrhea

Ingest 2-4 drops; massage 1-3 drops into abdomen clockwise hourly as needed.

Digestive Blend ^{T I}
Lemon ^{T I}
Ginger ^{T I}
Lavender ^{T I}
Spearmint ^{T I}

Diverticulitis

Ingest 2-4 drops twice daily for ongoing support; massage 1-3 drops into abdomen clockwise as needed.

Digestive Blend [TI]
Cypress [TI]
Lemon [TI]
Cellular Complex [TI]
Digestive Enzymes [I]

Dizziness

Apply 1-3 drops to back of neck, under nose, or on temples; inhale from cupped hands; ingest 2-4 drops of Detoxification Blend as needed.

Grounding Blend [AT]
Detoxification Blend [ATI]
Cypress [AT]
Cedarwood [AT]
Arborvitae [AT]

Drug Addiction

Apply a couple drops to chest, temples, and bottoms of feet daily; inhale from cupped hands as needed.

Copaiba [ATI]
Detoxification Blend [ATI]
Cleansing Blend [AT]
Black Pepper [ATI]
Frankincense [ATI]

Dysentery

Massage 1-3 drops into abdomen; ingest 2-4 drops as needed.

Helichrysum [TI]
Digestive Blend [TI]
Frankincense [TI]
Lavender [TI]
Melaleuca [TI]

Dysphagia

Apply 1-3 drops to neck or ingest a few drops as needed.

Copaiba [TI]
Marjoram [TI]
Lemon [TI]
Peppermint [TI]
Frankincense [TI]

Ear Infection

Apply 1-3 drops around the opening of the ear or apply to a cotton ball and place over ear opening overnight. Do NOT use essential oils in ear. Ingest 2-4 drops as needed.

Melaleuca [TI]
Lavender [TI]
Basil [TI]
Helichrysum [TI]
Melaleuca [TI]

Earache

Apply 1-3 drops around the opening of the ear or apply to a cotton ball and place over ear opening overnight. Do NOT use essential oils in ear.

Helichrysum [T]
Basil [T]
Lavender [T]
Melaleuca [T]
Frankincense [T]

Eczema

Apply 2-4 drops to affected area as needed. For improved efficacy, dilute with carrier oil.

Skin Clearing Blend [T]
Helichrysum [T]
Cedarwood [T]
Anti-Aging Blend [T]
Magnolia [T]
Protocol on pg. 171

Edema

Massage 2-4 drops into affected area and on bottoms of feet; ingest a couple times daily or as needed.

Lemon [TI]
Eucalyptus [TI]
Peppermint [TI]
Metabolic Blend [TI]
Grapefruit [TI]

Emphysema

Apply 1-3 drops to back of neck, under nose, chest, or on bridge of nose as needed; ingest 3-5 drops; inhale from cupped hands.

Respiratory Blend [AT]
Frankincense [ATI]
Rose [AT]
Eucalyptus [AT]
Lavender [ATI]

Energy (low)

Apply 2-4 drops to bottoms of feet, under nose, on bridge of nose, or chest as needed; inhale from cupped hands as needed.

Wild Orange [ATI]
Peppermint [ATI]
Spearmint [ATI]
Energy & Stamina Complex [I]
Vitality Trio [I]
Protocol on pg. 163

Epilepsy

Apply 1-3 drops to back of neck, under nose, or on temples; inhale from cupped hands; ingest 2-4 drops of Frankincense or Cellular Complex blend 3-5x daily.

Frankincense [ATI]
Spikenard [ATI]
Copaiba [ATI]
Cellular Complex [ATI]
Vitality Trio [I]

Erectile Dysfunction

Apply 2-4 drops to temples, wrists, and back of neck as needed; inhale from cupped hands; add a drop to personal lubricant.

Rose [AT]
Ylang Ylang [AT]
Inspiring Blend [AT]
Ginger [AT]
Cellular Complex [AT]

Estrogen Imbalance

Apply 2-4 drops to feet, abdomen, and lower back; inhale from cupped hands; take 2-4 drops of Clary Sage in a capsule 2x daily.

Clary Sage [ATI]
Lavender [ATI]
Basil [ATI]
Women's Perfume Blend [AT]
Phytoestrogen Complex [I]

Exhaustion

Inhale 1-3 drops from cupped hands; apply a couple drops to feet and back; ingest 2-4 drops Ylang Ylang or Tangerine as needed.

Ylang Ylang [ATI]
Tangerine [ATI]
Uplifting Blend [AT]
Encouraging Blend [AT]
Peppermint [ATI]

Eyes (Swollen)

Apply 1-3 drops around eyes (do not get directly in eyes).

Geranium [T]
Frankincense [T]
Rose [T]
Eucalyptus [T]
Juniper Berry [T]

Fainting

Inhale 1-3 drops from cupped hands as needed; apply a drop onto ears and under nose; diffuse several drops.

Peppermint [AT]
Frankincense [AT]
Wild Orange [AT]
Neroli [AT]
Respiratory Blend [AT]

Fear

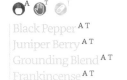

Inhale from cupped hands; apply a couple drops to feet and back.

Black Pepper [AT]
Juniper Berry [AT]
Grounding Blend [AT]
Frankincense [AT]
Encouraging Blend [AT]

Fever

Apply 2-4 drops to back of neck, under nose, on bridge of nose, or chest; ingest 2-4 drops Oregano every 2-4 hours until symptoms subside.

Peppermint [ATI]
Oregano [ATI]
Roman Chamomile [ATI]
Lavender [ATI]
Frankincense [ATI]

Fibrocystic Breasts

Massage 1-3 drops into breasts as needed; ingest 3-5 drops 3x daily.

Frankincense [TI]
Clary Sage [TI]
Sandalwood [TI]
Rose [T]
Cellular Complex [TI]

Fibroids (Uterine)

Apply 2-4 drops to abdomen 3x daily; ingest 3-5 drops.

Sandalwood [TI]
Thyme [TI]
Frankincense [TI]
Cellular Complex [TI]
Helichrysum [TI]

Fibromyalgia

Apply 2-4 drops to affected area; ingest 2-4 drops 3x daily; use full protocol for most profound results.

Cellular Complex [ATI]
Soothing Blend [AT]
Copaiba [ATI]
Frankincense [ATI]
Turmeric [ATI]
Protocol on pg. 172

Flu (Influenza)

Apply 2-4 drops to chest, bottoms of feet, and back over lungs; ingest 2-4 drops every 2-3 hours as desired for antiviral and immune-boosting support.

Respiratory Blend [AT]
Protective Blend [ATI]
Oregano [ATI]
Thyme [ATI]
Black Pepper [ATI]
Protocol on pg. 172

Focus & Concentration

Apply 1-3 drops to forehead, temples, back of neck, and behind the ears; inhale from cupped hands; diffuse several drops.

Peppermint [AT]
Focus Blend [AT]
Rosemary [AT]
Frankincense [AT]
Green Mandarin [AT]
Protocol on pg. 161

27

Food Poisoning

Apply 1-3 drops to stomach and rub clockwise; ingest 2-4 drops every 2-4 hours as needed.

Oregano ᵀ ᴵ
Digestive Blend ᵀ ᴵ
Pink Pepper ᵀ ᴵ
Protective Blend ᵀ ᴵ
GI Cleansing Complex ᴵ

Frozen Shoulder

Apply 2-4 drops to affected area. Massage with carrier oil for improved efficacy.

Soothing Blend ᵀ
Massage Blend ᵀ
Cypress ᵀ
Siberian Fir ᵀ
Lemongrass ᵀ

Fungal Skin

Apply 1-3 drops to affected area several times daily.

Melaleuca ᵀ
Skin Clearing Blend ᵀ
Oregano ᵀ
Arborvitae ᵀ
Cedarwood ᵀ

Gallbladder Issues

Massage 2-4 drops over gallbladder several times daily; ingest 2-4 drops as needed.

Juniper Berry ᵀ ᴵ
Detoxification Blend ᵀ ᴵ
Melaleuca ᵀ ᴵ
Helichrysum ᵀ ᴵ
Tangerine ᵀ ᴵ

Gallbladder Stones

Apply 2-4 drops over gallbladder several times daily; ingest 2-4 drops as needed.

Lemon ᵀ ᴵ
Cilantro ᵀ ᴵ
Rosemary ᵀ ᴵ
Bergamot ᵀ ᴵ
Detoxification Blend ᵀ ᴵ

Gas (Flatulence)

Massage 1-3 drops into stomach area; ingest 1-3 drops as needed.

Digestive Blend ᵀ ᴵ
Fennel ᵀ ᴵ
Peppermint ᵀ ᴵ
Ginger ᵀ ᴵ
Tangerine ᵀ ᴵ
Protocol on pg. 170

Gastritis

Massage 1-3 drops into stomach area; ingest 2-4 drops diluted in carrier oil inside a veggie cap as needed.

Lavender ᵀ ᴵ
Peppermint ᵀ ᴵ
Roman Chamomile ᵀ ᴵ
Lemon ᵀ ᴵ
Coriander ᵀ ᴵ
Protocol on pg. 171

Genital Warts

Dilute heavily with a carrier oil and apply 1-3 drops to affected area 3x daily.

Oregano ᵀ
Frankincense ᵀ
Melissa ᵀ
Melaleuca ᵀ
Lemon ᵀ

28

Giardia

Massage 1-3 drops clockwise onto stomach and chest area; ingest 1-3 drops as needed.

Digestive Blend [T I]
Oregano [T I]
Rosemary [T I]
Spearmint [T I]
Melaleuca [T I]

Gingivitis

Gargle 1-3 drops mixed with water several times daily; ingest 1-3 drops as needed.

Protective Blend [I]
Myrrh [I]
Clove [I]
Melaleuca [I]
Arborvitae [T]

Gluten Sensitivity

Ingest 1-3 drops as needed. Ingest digestive enzymes 20-30 minutes before eating, or immediately after or during consumption. Rub 2-4 drops over stomach.

Digestive Enzymes [I]
Digestive Blend [T I]
Lemon [T I]
Detoxification Blend [T I]
Seasonal Blend [T I]

Gout

Ingest 2-4 drops twice a day; massage 1-3 drops gently into affected joints as needed.

Lemongrass [T I]
Birch [T]
Soothing Blend [T]
Peppermint [T I]
Lavender [T I]
Protocol on pg. 163

Growing Pains

Massage 2-4 drops into affected areas as needed.

Soothing Blend [T]
Marjoram [T]
Lemongrass [T]
Wintergreen [T]
Spikenard [T]

Gum Disease

Apply 1-3 drops to gums, gargle a few drops in water as needed.

Protective blend [I]
Myrrh [I]
Clove [I]
Melaleuca [I]
Lavender [I]

Gums (Bleeding)

Apply 1-3 drops to gums; gargle a few drops in water as needed.

Helichrysum [I]
Myrrh [I]
Geranium [I]
Melaleuca [I]
Clove [I]

Hair Loss

Dilute 5 drops in 20 drops of carrier oil. Massage into scalp every night or 30 minutes before showering.

Rosemary [T]
Peppermint [T]
Geranium [T]
Spikenard [T]
Vitality Trio [I]

Halitosis

Gargle a few drops mixed with water several times daily or as needed; ingest 1-3 drops Cilantro twice daily.

Protective Blend [I]
Cilantro [I]
Peppermint [I]
Detoxification Blend [I]
Spearmint [I]

Hand, Foot, & Mouth

Apply 1-3 drops to affected areas (dilute for increased effectiveness); ingest as needed.

Protective Blend [TI]
Rose [TI]
Cellular Complex [TI]
Copaiba [TI]
Melissa [TI]

Hangover

Add 4-6 drops to warm bath; massage into back of neck and over liver; ingest 2-4 drops as needed.

Digestive Blend [ATI]
Tension Blend [ATI]
Grapefruit [ATI]
Detoxification Blend [ATI]
Lemon [ATI]

Hay Fever

Apply 1-3 drops to bridge of nose and over sinuses or chest as needed; use a drop of Lavender under the tongue; inhale from cupped hands; diffuse several drops.

Respiratory Blend [AT]
Lavender [ATI]
Peppermint [ATI]
Cleansing Blend [AT]
Seasonal Blend [I]
Protocol on pg. 162

Head Lice

Dilute 1-3 drops and apply to entire scalp, shampoo, and rinse 30 minutes later. Repeat daily for several days.

Melaleuca [T]
Arborvitae [T]
Outdoor Blend [T]
Rosemary [T]
Eucalyptus [T]

Headache

Massage 1-3 drops into forehead, temples, and back of neck; inhale from cupped hands.

Tension Blend [AT]
Peppermint [AT]
Frankincense [AT]
Lavender [AT]
Massage Blend [AT]

Hearing Issues

Apply 1-3 drops to temples and around the opening of the ear; apply to a cotton ball and place over ear opening overnight. Do not apply into ear.

Helichrysum [T]
Basil [T]
Frankincense [T]
Rose [T]
Melaleuca [T]

Heart Disease

  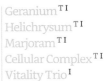

Apply 2-4 drops over chest; ingest 3-5 drops as a daily supplement.

Geranium [TI]
Helichrysum [TI]
Marjoram [TI]
Cellular Complex [TI]
Vitality Trio [I]

Heartburn

Massage 1-3 drops into abdomen; ingest 1-3 drops as needed.

Digestive Blend [TI]
Peppermint [TI]
Metabolic Blend [TI]
Ginger [TI]
Fennel [TI]
Protocol on pg. 172

Heat Exhaustion

Apply 1-3 drops to forehead, back of neck, inside of wrists, and bottom of feet; add Lemon or Peppermint to mineral water and sip slowly.

Peppermint [ATI]
Lemon [ATI]
Tension Blend [AT]
Siberian Fir [ATI]
Lavender [ATI]

Heatstroke

Apply 1-3 drops to forehead, temples, back of neck, and chest; ingest 1-3 drops as needed.

Peppermint [ATI]
Frankincense [ATI]
Tension Blend [AT]
Spearmint [ATI]
Copaiba [ATI]

Heavy Metal Detox

Ingest 2-4 drops 2x daily; massage 2-4 drops into bottoms of feet.

Cilantro [TI]
Frankincense [TI]
Cellular Complex [TI]
Detox Herbal Complex [I]
Lemon [TI]

Hematoma

Apply 1-3 drops to affected areas 2-3x daily or as needed; take 3-5 drops in a capsule 2x daily.

Cypress [T]
Massage Blend [T]
Geranium [TI]
Marjoram [TI]
Lemon [TI]

Hemorrhoids

Dilute 2-4 drops with carrier oil and apply directly to affected areas daily or as needed.

Geranium [T]
Cypress [T]
Rose [T]
Siberian Fir [T]
Myrrh [T]

Hepatitis

Ingest 1-3 drops; use several drops topically with a warm compress over the liver area.

Copaiba [TI]
Myrrh [TI]
Detoxification Blend [TI]
Helichrysum [TI]
Lavender [TI]

Hernia (hiatal)

Massage 1-3 drops into affected area as needed.

Helichrysum [T]
Frankincense [T]
Arborvitae [T]
Digestive Blend [T]
Digestive Enzymes [I]

Ailments

31

Herniated Disc

Massage 2-4 drops into affected area as often as needed (at least 3x daily).

Soothing Blend [T]
Massage Blend [T]
Lemongrass [T]
Copaiba [T]
Wintergreen [T]

Herpes Simplex

Ingest 1-3 drops; use topically with a warm compress over the kidney area; apply on the right and left side of throat daily.

Melaleuca [T I]
Melissa [T I]
Protective Blend [T I]
Oregano [T I]
Rose [T]

Hiccups

Inhale 1-3 drops from cupped hands; massage into chest and stomach area as needed.

Arborvitae [A T]
Lemon [A T]
Copaiba [A T]
Digestive Blend [A T]
Neroli [A T]

HIV

Apply 1-3 drops to bottoms of feet; ingest 3-5 drops 3x daily; inhale from cupped hands for emotional support.

Melissa [A T I]
Oregano [A T I]
Helichrysum [A T I]
Cellular Complex [A T I]
Thyme [A T I]
Protocol on pg. 161

Hives

Apply 1-3 drops diluted to affected area; ingest 2-4 drops twice daily as needed.

Melaleuca [T I]
Frankincense [T I]
Lavender [T I]
Men's Blend [T]
Magnolia [T]

Hoarse Voice

Gargle 1-3 drops in water as needed; apply diluted to outside of throat.

Lemon [T I]
Myrrh [T I]
Lavender [T I]
Protective Blend [T I]
Arborvitae [T]

Hormone Balance

Massage 2-4 drops into abdomen, temples, and bottoms of feet; ingest as needed; inhale from cupped hands.

Women's Monthly Blend [A T]
Clary Sage [A T I]
Ylang Ylang [A T I]
Frankincense [A T I]
Sandalwood [A T I]

Hot Flashes

Massage 2-4 drops into chest, neck, and face as needed; ingest 2-5 drops Clary Sage and Ylang Ylang 2x daily.

Women's Monthly Blend [A T]
Peppermint [A T I]
Clary Sage [A T I]
Ylang Ylang [A T I]
Women's Perfume Blend [A T]
Protocol on pg. 175

Hyperactivity

Apply 1-3 drops on back of neck and bottoms of feet; inhale from cupped hands; diffuse several drops.

Focus Blend ᴬ ᵀ
Grounding Blend ᴬ ᵀ
Vetiver ᴬ ᵀ
Frankincense ᴬ ᵀ
Lavender ᴬ ᵀ

Hypertension

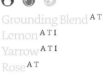

Apply 1-2 drops behind ears; inhale from cupped hands; use a drop under the tongue; diffuse several drops.

Grounding Blend ᴬ ᵀ
Lemon ᴬ ᵀ ᴵ
Yarrow ᴬ ᵀ ᴵ
Rose ᴬ ᵀ
Manuka ᴬ ᵀ
Protocol on pg. 179

Hyperthyroid

Apply 1-3 drops to front of neck. Dilute with carrier oil for easier application. Ingest 3-5 drops a few times daily or as needed.

Myrrh ᵀ ᴵ
Frankincense ᵀ ᴵ
Cellular Complex ᵀ ᴵ
Detoxification Blend ᵀ ᴵ
Vitality Trio ᴵ
Protocol on pg. 180

Hypoglycemia

Apply 1-3 drops to chest, bottoms of feet, and inside of wrists; ingest 2-4 drops a few times daily or as needed.

Metabolic Blend ᵀ ᴵ
Cinnamon ᵀ ᴵ
Coriander ᵀ ᴵ
Detoxification Blend ᵀ ᴵ
Cellular Complex ᵀ ᴵ

Hypothyroid

Apply 1-3 drops to front of neck. Dilute with carrier oil for easier application. Ingest 3-5 drops a few times daily or as needed.

Peppermint ᵀ ᴵ
Lemongrass ᵀ ᴵ
Clove ᵀ ᴵ
Myrrh ᵀ ᴵ
Vitality Trio ᴵ
Protocol on pg. 181

Immune Boost

Apply 2-4 drops to bottoms of feet; ingest 3-5 drops 2x daily; inhale from cupped hands as needed

Protective Blend ᴬ ᵀ ᴵ
Melaleuca ᴬ ᵀ ᴵ
Oregano ᴬ ᵀ ᴵ
Black Pepper ᴬ ᵀ ᴵ
Clove ᴬ ᵀ ᴵ
Protocol on pg. 173

Indigestion

Massage 1-3 drops into stomach area clockwise as needed; drink 1-3 drops with water or in a capsule.

Digestive Blend ᵀ ᴵ
Ginger ᵀ ᴵ
Lemon ᵀ ᴵ
Cardamom ᵀ ᴵ
Digestive Tablets ᴵ
Protocol on pg. 171

Infant Reflux

Apply 1-2 drops diluted to stomach area and chest as needed.

Digestive Blend ᵀ
Lavender ᵀ
Fennel ᵀ
Frankincense ᵀ
Ginger ᵀ

Ailments

33

Infected Wounds

Apply 1-3 drops to affected areas 2-3x daily as needed; dilute for sensitive skin.

Melaleuca [T]
Helichrysum [T]
Frankincense [T]
Lavender [T]
Protective Blend [T]

Infertility

Apply 2-4 drops to abdomen, wrists, and lower back daily; ingest 2-4 drops 2x daily.

Clary Sage [A T I]
Cellular Complex [A T I]
Ylang Ylang [A T I]
Fennel [A T I]
Vitality Trio [I]
Protocol on pg. 173

Inflammation

Apply 2-4 drops to affected areas as needed. For systemic inflammation, ingest 2-4 drops 2x daily.

Soothing Blend [A T]
Frankincense [A T I]
Copaiba [A T I]
Turmeric [A T I]
Wintergreen [A T]

Inflammatory Bowel Disease

Massage 1-3 drops onto stomach; ingest 2-4 drops 2-3x daily.

Digestive Blend [T I]
Frankincense [T I]
Lavender [T I]
Digestive Enzymes [I]
Probiotic Complex [I]
Protocol on pg. 173

Ingrown Toenail

Apply 1-3 drops to affected toenail 3x daily.

Melaleuca [T]
Protective Blend [T]
Detoxification Blend [T]
Lavender [T]
Oregano [T]

Insect Bites

Apply 1-2 drops to insect bite hourly or as needed.

Lavender [T]
Melaleuca [T]
Cleansing Blend [T]
Roman Chamomile [T]
Frankincense [T]

Insomnia

Apply 1-3 drops to forehead, temples, base of skull, and behind the ear; diffuse several drops.

Restful Blend [A T]
Vetiver [A T]
Lavender [A T]
Cedarwood [A T]
Petitgrain [A T]
Protocol on pg. 178

Insulin Imbalance

Apply 2-4 drops to bottoms of feet; take 3-5 drops internally 2x daily.

Cinnamon [T I]
Protective Blend [T I]
Lavender [T I]
Clove [T I]
Metabolic Blend [T I]
Protocol on pg. 170

Ailments

Irritable Bowel Syndrome

Apply 1-3 drops to bottoms of feet or over stomach; take 2-4 drops internally as needed.

Digestive Blend ᵀ ¹
Ginger ᵀ ¹
Turmeric ᵀ ¹
Frankincense ᵀ ¹
Peppermint ᵀ ¹
Protocol on pg. 173

Itchy Skin

Apply 1-3 drops to affected areas as needed. Use with carrier oil or lotion for improved efficacy.

Melaleuca ᵀ
Lavender ᵀ
Skin Clearing Blend ᵀ
Cedarwood ᵀ
Frankincense ᵀ
Protocol on pg. 171

Jaundice

Massage 1-3 drops diluted over the liver; diffuse several drops nearby.

Lavender ᴬ ᵀ
Myrrh ᴬ ᵀ
Neroli ᴬ ᵀ
Rose ᴬ ᵀ
Grapefruit ᴬ ᵀ

Jet Lag

Apply 1-3 drops to forehead, temples, back of neck, and chest; inhale from cupped hands as needed.

Peppermint ᴬ ᵀ
Tangerine ᴬ ᵀ
Lemon ᴬ ᵀ
Protective Blend ᴬ ᵀ
Cellular Complex ᴬ ᵀ

Jock Itch

Apply 1-3 drops to affected areas as needed with carrier oil; ingest 3-4 drops 3x daily.

Melaleuca ᵀ ¹
Skin Clearing Blend ᵀ
Lavender ᵀ ¹
Cleansing Blend ᵀ
Thyme ᵀ ¹

Joint Pain

Massage 1-3 drops into affected areas as needed; use carrier oil for improved efficacy.

Soothing Blend ᵀ
Lemongrass ᵀ
Wintergreen ᵀ
Copaiba ᵀ
Frankincense ᵀ
Protocol on pg. 163

Kidney Infection

Apply 2-4 drops over kidneys 3-5x daily; ingest 1-3 drops 3-5x daily.

Juniper Berry ᵀ ¹
Lemongrass ᵀ ¹
Oregano ᵀ ¹
Protective Blend ᵀ ¹
Clove ᵀ ¹

Kidney Stones

Massage 2-4 drops over kidneys 3-5x daily; ingest 1-3 drops 3-5x daily.

Lemon ᵀ ¹
Juniper Berry ᵀ ¹
Helichrysum ᵀ ¹
Wintergreen ᵀ
Wild Orange ᵀ ¹

Lactose Intolerance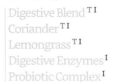

Ingest 2-4 drops or massage over stomach as needed.

Digestive Blend ^{T I}
Coriander ^{T I}
Lemongrass ^{T I}
Digestive Enzymes ^I
Probiotic Complex ^I

Laryngitis

Diffuse several drops throughout the day; ingest 3-5 drops 3x daily; massage 1-3 drops onto outside of throat.

Protective Blend ^{A T I}
Melaleuca ^{A T I}
Pink Pepper ^{A T I}
Lemon ^{A T I}
Rosemary ^{A T I}

Leg Cramps

Massage several drops into legs as needed; use carrier oil for improved efficacy.

Soothing Blend ^T
Cypress ^T
Massage Blend ^T
Marjoram ^T
Black Pepper ^T

Leukemia

Ingest 2-4 drops 3x daily; massage 2-4 drops into bottoms of feet and spine 3-5x daily.

Cellular Complex ^{T I}
Frankincense ^{T I}
Lemongrass ^{T I}
Sandalwood ^{T I}
Myrrh ^{T I}

Libido (low)

Apply 1-3 drops to abdomen, bottoms of feet, and wrists as needed; inhale from cupped hands; diffuse several drops.

Inspiring Blend ^{A T}
Ylang Ylang ^{A T}
Jasmine ^{A T}
Women's Monthly Blend ^{A T}
Rose ^{A T}
Protocol on pg. 174

Lupus

Ingest 2-4 drops 3-5x daily during flare ups; massage 2-4 drops into inflamed areas; diffuse several drops for emotional support.

Frankincense ^{A T I}
Cellular Complex ^{A T I}
Soothing Blend ^{A T}
Copaiba ^{A T I}
Turmeric ^{A T I}
Protocol on pg. 174

Lyme Disease

Massage 2-4 drops into lower back 3x daily; take 3-5 drops in a capsule 3x daily.

Melissa ^{T I}
Thyme ^{T I}
Oregano ^{T I}
Geranium ^{T I}
Vitality Trio ^I
Protocol on pg. 174

Measles

Dab a few drops onto spots several times daily; add several drops to bath and soak for at least 30 minutes as needed.

Lavender ^T
Roman Chamomile ^T
Oregano ^T
Eucalyptus ^T
Protective Blend ^T

Melanoma

Apply 2-4 drops to affected areas 3-5x daily; ingest 2-4 drops 3x daily.

Frankincense ᵀ ᴵ
Cellular Complex ᵀ ᴵ
Sandalwood ᵀ ᴵ
Rose ᵀ
Clove ᵀ ᴵ

Memory Loss

Massage 2-4 drops into forehead, temples, back of neck, and chest as needed; inhale from cupped hands.

Rosemary ᴬ ᵀ
Peppermint ᴬ ᵀ
Bergamot ᴬ ᵀ
Lavender ᴬ ᵀ
Frankincense ᴬ ᵀ

Meningitis

Ingest 2-4 drops 2x daily; massage 2-4 drops into back of neck with carrier oil daily.

Protective Blend ᵀ ᴵ
Lavender ᵀ ᴵ
Oregano ᵀ ᴵ
Melissa ᵀ ᴵ
Cellular Complex ᵀ ᴵ

Menopause

Apply 2-4 drops topically to abdomen, bottoms of feet, and back of neck daily; ingest 2-4 drops Clary Sage and Siberian Fir as needed.

Clary Sage ᵀ ᴵ
Women's Monthly Blend ᵀ
Siberian Fir ᵀ ᴵ
Geranium ᵀ ᴵ
Cellular Complex ᵀ ᴵ
Protocol on pg. 175

Menstrual Bleeding

Massage 2-4 drops into abdomen and lower back; apply to a warm compress over uterus area; ingest 2-4 drops as needed.

Helichrysum ᵀ ᴵ
Geranium ᵀ ᴵ
Clary Sage ᵀ ᴵ
Women's Monthly Blend ᵀ
Lavender ᵀ ᴵ

Menstrual Pain

Massage 1-3 drops into abdomen, lower back, and shoulders; apply to a warm compress over uterus area; ingest 2-4 drops as needed.

Women's Monthly Blend ᵀ
Frankincense ᴬ ᵀ ᴵ
Peppermint ᴬ ᵀ ᴵ
Clary Sage ᴬ ᵀ ᴵ
Marjoram ᴬ ᵀ ᴵ
Protocol on pg. 175

Mental Fatigue

Massage 1-3 drops into forehead, temples, back of neck, and bottoms of feet; inhale from cupped hands as needed.

Peppermint ᴬ ᵀ
Basil ᴬ ᵀ
Green Mandarin ᴬ ᵀ
Frankincense ᴬ ᵀ
Energy & Stamina Complex ᴵ

Migraine

Apply 1-3 drops to forehead, temples, base of skull, back of neck, and bottoms of feet; inhale from cupped hands as needed.

Tension Blend ᴬ ᵀ
Peppermint ᴬ ᵀ
Frankincense ᴬ ᵀ
Soothing Blend ᴬ ᵀ
Copaiba ᴬ ᵀ

Mold & Mildew

Diffuse several drops where mold is present throughout the day until no longer needed. Mix 20 drops with 4 oz water and apply to area of concern.

Melaleuca [T]
Cleansing Blend [T]
Protective Blend [T]
Oregano [T]
Lemon [T]

Moles

Apply a drop to mole 2-3x daily (avoid surrounding skin with hot oils like Oregano).

Oregano [T]
Frankincense [T]
Cellular Complex [T]
Skin Clearing Blend [T]
Cleansing Blend [T]

Mononucleosis

Ingest 3-5 drops 3x daily; apply 2-4 drops to bottoms of feet; diffuse several drops.

Digestive Blend [A T I]
Peppermint [A T I]
Ginger [A T I]
Fennel [A T I]
Coriander [A T I]
Protocol on pg. 175

Mood Swings

Inhale 1-3 drops from cupped hands; apply a few drops to forehead, temples, back of neck, and bottoms of feet; diffuse several drops.

Grounding Blend [A T]
Uplifting Blend [A T]
Frankincense [A T]
Lime [A T]
Wild Orange [A T]

Morning Sickness

Apply 1-3 drops behind ears and over navel hourly; inhale from cupped hands; ingest 1-3 drops as needed.

Ginger [A T I]
Peppermint [A T I]
Digestive Blend [A T I]
Fennel [A T I]
Coriander [A T I]
Protocol on pg. 176

Motion Sickness

Apply 1-3 drops behind the ears and over navel; inhale from cupped hands; use a drop under the tongue.

Digestive Blend [A T I]
Peppermint [A T I]
Ginger [A T I]
Grounding Blend [A T]
Basil [A T I]

Mouth Ulcers

Gargle 1-3 drops mixed with water several times daily; apply a dab to affected area 2-3x daily.

Protective Blend [T I]
Clove [T I]
Myrrh [T I]
Sandalwood [T I]
Melaleuca [T I]

Muscle Injury

Massage 2-4 drops into affected muscles 3x daily or as needed.

Soothing Blend [T]
Marjoram [T]
Helichrysum [T]
Massage Blend [T]
Yarrow [T]
Protocol on pg. 176

Ailments

Muscle Pain

Massage 2-4 drops into affected muscles 3x daily or as needed; use a drop under the tongue for pain relief.

Soothing Blend [T]
Marjoram [T]
Helichrysum [T]
Massage Blend [T]
Copaiba [T I]

Protocol on pg. 176

Muscle Spasms

Massage 2-4 drops into affected muscles as needed; use a drop under the tongue.

Black Pepper [T I]
Soothing Blend [T]
Copaiba [T I]
Blue Tansy [T]
Yarrow [T I]

Muscle Stiffness

Massage 2-4 drops into affected muscles 2-3x daily.

Massage Blend [T]
Soothing Blend [T]
Cypress [T]
Lemongrass [T]
Marjoram [T]

Protocol on pg. 168

Nasal Congestion

Apply 1-3 drops over bridge of nose, under nose, and rub over sinuses; diffuse several drops.

Respiratory Blend [A T]
Siberian Fir [A T]
Lime [A T]
Eucalyptus [A T]
Peppermint [A T]

Nasal Polyps

Apply 1-3 drops over bridge of nose and under nose.

Frankincense [T]
Melaleuca [T]
Melissa [T]
Respiratory Blend [T]
Oregano [T]

Nausea

Apply 1-3 drops behind ears and over navel hourly; use a drop under the tongue; inhale from cupped hands.

Digestive Blend [A T I]
Ginger [A T I]
Peppermint [A T I]
Cardamom [A T I]
Grounding Blend [A T]

Neck Pain

Massage 2-4 drops onto neck several times daily; use carrier oil to improve efficacy; use a drop of Copaiba under the tongue for pain.

Soothing Blend [A T]
Lemongrass [A T]
Copaiba [A T I]
Wintergreen [A T]
Douglas Fir [A T]

Protocol on pg. 164

Nervous Fatigue

Inhale from cupped hands; apply 1-3 drops to temples, behind ears, and on back of neck as needed; diffuse several drops.

Grounding Blend [A T]
Lemon [A T]
Cedarwood [A T]
Vetiver [A T]
Tangerine [A T]

Neuropathy

Apply 2-4 drops to affected areas several times daily; ingest 1-3 drops as needed.

Soothing Blend [T]
Frankincense [T I]
Massage Blend [T]
Roman Chamomile [T I]
Peppermint [T I]

Night Sweats

Apply 2-4 drops to abdomen and back of neck before sleeping.

Detoxification Blend [T]
Cellular Complex [T]
Peppermint [T]
Lavender [T]
Lime [T]

Nightmares

Apply 2-4 drops to abdomen and back of neck before sleeping; diffuse several drops.

Juniper Berry [A T]
Restful Blend [A T]
Cedarwood [A T]
Lavender [A T]
Reassuring Blend [A T]

Nosebleeds

Apply 1-3 drops to the bridge and sides of nose and back of neck as needed.

Helichrysum [T]
Geranium [T]
Frankincense [T]
Lavender [T]
Cypress [T]

Odors

Diffuse several drops; apply 2-3 drops with a carrier oil to surface odors; ingest 3-5 drops twice daily for body odors.

Cleansing Blend [A T]
Melaleuca [A T I]
Cilantro [A T I]
Lemon [A T I]
Douglas Fir [A T]

Osteoarthritis

Massage 2-4 drops into affected areas daily; use carrier oil for improved efficacy.

Soothing Blend [T]
Frankincense [T]
Lemongrass [T]
Copaiba [T]
Cellular Complex [T]

Osteoporosis

Massage 2-4 drops onto spine and affected areas daily; take 2-4 drops Cellular Complex internally 2x daily.

Wintergreen [T]
Birch [T]
Frankincense [T I]
Cellular Complex [T I]
Bone Nutrient [I]

Ovarian Cysts

Blend 1-3 drops with carrier oil and soak tampon to insert overnight; apply 3-5 drops with warm compress over abdomen; take 3-5 drops internally.

Frankincense [T I]
Clary Sage [T I]
Cellular Complex [T I]
Oregano [T I]
Sandalwood [T I]

Overeating

Apply 1-3 drops to stomach; take 2-4 drops internally; inhale from cupped hands as needed.

Metabolic Blend ^{A T I}
Peppermint ^{A T I}
Grapefruit ^{A T I}
Renewing Blend ^{A T}
Cinnamon ^{A T I}
Protocol on pg. 181

Palpitations

Apply 1-3 drops over heart 3x daily; inhale from cupped hands.

Marjoram ^{A T}
Lavender ^{A T}
Geranium ^{A T}
Ylang Ylang ^{A T}
Wild Orange ^{A T}

Pancreatitis

Ingest 1-3 drops 3x daily; massage 1-3 drops over abdomen as needed.

Detoxification Blend ^{T I}
Marjoram ^{T I}
Lemon ^{T I}
Coriander ^{T I}
Rosemary ^{T I}

Parasites

Ingest 3-5 drops 3x daily; apply in a warm compress over intestinal area 2-3x daily.

Detoxification Blend ^{T I}
Oregano ^{T I}
Geranium ^{T I}
Clove ^{T I}
Thyme ^{T I}
Protocol on pg. 170

Pink Eye
(Conjunctivitis)

Apply 1-2 drops around (but not in) eyes 3x daily; dilute for sensitive skin.

Melaleuca ^T
Rosemary ^T
Arborvitae ^T
Clary Sage ^T
Cleansing Blend ^T

Plantar Warts

Apply 1-3 drops to wart several times daily (avoid surrounding skin with hot oils like Oregano.)

Oregano ^T
Frankincense ^T
Cellular Complex ^T
Melissa ^T
Rose ⁱ

Pneumonia

Apply 2-4 drops to chest, neck, and bottoms of feet 3-5x daily; gargle a drop hourly; inhale from cupped hands as needed; diffuse several drops.

Respiratory Blend ^{A T}
Protective Blend ^{A T I}
Arborvitae ^{A T}
Bergamot ^{A T I}
Roman Chamomile ^{A T I}
Protocol on pg. 165

Poison Ivy/Oak

Apply 1-3 drops to affected area with carrier oil a couple times daily or as needed.

Lavender ^T
Frankincense ^T
Geranium ^T
Patchouli ^T
Petitgrain ^T

Ailments

41

Post Traumatic Stress Disorder

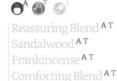

Apply 2-4 drops to forehead, temples, back of neck, chest, and bottoms of feet; inhale from cupped hands as needed.

Reassuring Blend ᴬ ᵀ
Sandalwood ᴬ ᵀ
Frankincense ᴬ ᵀ
Comforting Blend ᴬ ᵀ
Renewing Blend ᴬ ᵀ

PMS

Add 3-6 drops to warm bath; apply to abdomen; inhale from cupped hands; ingest 1-3 drops as needed.

Women's Monthly Blend ᴬ ᵀ
Clary Sage ᴬ ᵀ ᴵ
Geranium ᴬ ᵀ ᴵ
Frankincense ᴬ ᵀ ᴵ
Women's Perfume Blend ᴬ ᵀ
Protocol on pg. 175

Prostatitis

Apply 3-5 drops to lower abdomen and lower back 3x daily or as needed.

Rosemary ᵀ
Marjoram ᵀ
Thyme ᵀ
Frankincense ᵀ
Myrrh ᵀ

Psoriasis

Apply 1-3 drops to affected area a couple times daily with carrier oil; ingest 2-4 drops 2x daily.

Melaleuca ᴬ ᵀ ᴵ
Detoxification Blend ᴬ ᵀ ᴵ
Thyme ᴬ ᵀ ᴵ
Roman Chamomile ᴬ ᵀ ᴵ
Probiotic Complex ᴵ
Protocol on pg. 177

Rashes

Dilute 1-3 drops with a carrier oil and apply to affected area as needed.

Melaleuca ᵀ
Roman Chamomile ᵀ
Lavender ᵀ
Cedarwood ᵀ
Magnolia ᵀ
Protocol on pg. 171

Respiratory Issues

Apply 2-4 drops to chest, neck, under nose, and on bridge of nose; inhale from cupped hands as needed; diffuse several drops.

Respiratory Blend ᴬ ᵀ
Eucalyptus ᴬ ᵀ
Douglas Fir ᴬ ᵀ
Cardamom ᴬ ᵀ
Rosemary ᴬ ᵀ

Restless Leg Syndrome

Massage 2-4 drops onto legs and bottoms of feet; diffuse several drops; use 2 drops Yarrow under the tongue.

Soothing Blend ᴬ ᵀ
Ylang Ylang ᴬ ᵀ
Cypress ᴬ ᵀ
Petitgrain ᴬ ᵀ
Yarrow ᴬ ᵀ ᴵ

Restlessness

Inhale 1-3 drops from cupped hands; apply 2-4 drops to bottoms of feet and back of neck as needed.

Grounding Blend ᴬ ᵀ
Lavender ᴬ ᵀ
Restful Blend ᴬ ᵀ
Vetiver ᴬ ᵀ
Spikenard ᴬ ᵀ

Rheumatic Fever

Apply 1-3 drops to bottoms of feet; ingest 1-3 drops twice daily; gargle a few drops mixed with water as needed.

Oregano [T I]
Peppermint [T I]
Melissa [T I]
Wintergreen [T]
Arborvitae [T]

Rhinitis

Inhale 1-3 drops from cupped hands several times daily; apply a couple drops to forehead and bridge of nose; ingest 2-4 drops 3x daily; diffuse several drops.

Respiratory Blend [A T]
Melaleuca [A T I]
Pink Pepper [A T I]
Siberian Fir [A T I]
Oregano [A T I]

Ringworm

Apply 1-3 drops to affected area 3-4x daily; use with carrier oil for improved efficacy; take 2-4 drops in a capsule 3x daily.

Melaleuca [T I]
Cleansing Blend [T]
Skin Clearing Blend [T]
Petitgrain [T I]
Detoxification Blend [T I]

Scarring

Massage 2-4 drops into scarred area 2x daily.

Anti-Aging Blend [T]
Frankincense [T]
Helichrysum [T]
Sandalwood [T]
Neroli [T]

Sciatica

Massage 1-3 drops into affected area a couple times daily.

Soothing Blend [T]
Frankincense [T]
Vetiver [T]
Copaiba [T]
Helichrysum [T]
Protocol on pg. 164

Seizures

Apply 1-3 drops to back of neck and bottoms of feet; inhale from cupped hands as needed; take 1-3 drops internally twice daily.

Spikenard [A T I]
Grounding Blend [A T]
Sandalwood [A T I]
Roman Chamomile [A T I]
Petitgrain [A T I]

Shingles

Apply 2-4 drops to affected areas, on back of neck, and along the spine 3x daily; take 2-4 drops 3x daily.

Melaleuca [T I]
Melissa [T I]
Black Pepper [T I]
Yarrow [T I]
Geranium [T I]
Protocol on pg. 177

Shock

Apply 1-3 drops on temples, under nose, and on back of neck as needed; inhale from cupped hands; diffuse several drops.

Grounding Blend [A T]
Frankincense [A T]
Helichrysum [A T]
Uplifting Blend [A T]
Renewing Blend [A T]

Sinus Infection

Apply 1-3 drops over bridge of nose and sinuses (avoid eyes) 3x daily; diffuse several drops; take 3-5 drops in a capsule 3x daily.

Black Pepper ᴬᵀᴵ
Grapefruit ᴬᵀᴵ
Basil ᴬᵀᴵ
Bergamot ᴬᵀᴵ
Detoxification Blend ᴬᵀᴵ
Protocol on pg. 177

Skin Ulcers

Apply 1-3 drops diluted into affected area 2-3x daily.

Lavender ᵀ
Myrrh ᵀ
Skin Clearing Blend ᵀ
Sandalwood ᵀ
Yarrow ᵀ

Smoking Addiction

Ingest 2-4 drops daily; inhale from cupped hands as needed when experiencing cravings.

Black Pepper ᴬᵀᴵ
Grapefruit ᴬᵀᴵ
Basil ᴬᵀᴵ
Bergamot ᴬᵀᴵ
Detoxification Blend ᴬᵀᴵ
Protocol on pg. 178

Snoring

Apply 1-3 drops to chest and under nose; diffuse several drops near bedside; gargle Protective Blend with water to open throat.

Respiratory Blend ᴬᵀ
Protective Blend ᴬᵀᴵ
Petitgrain ᴬᵀ
Eucalyptus ᴬᵀ
Douglas Fir ᴬᵀ
Protocol on pg. 179

Sore Throat

Gargle 1-3 drops with water, then swallow; apply to throat and neck, diluting with carrier oil as needed.

Protective Blend ᵀᴵ
Oregano ᵀᴵ
Lemon ᵀᴵ
Arborvitae ᵀ
Melissa ᵀᴵ
Protocol on pg. 179

Sprains

Gently apply 2-4 drops to affected area as needed.

Soothing Blend ᵀ
Helichrysum ᵀ
Lemongrass ᵀ
Spikenard ᵀ
Massage Blend ᵀ

Stomach Ache

Rub 2-4 drops over stomach as needed; ingest 1-3 drops as needed.

Digestive Blend ᵀᴵ
Ginger ᵀᴵ
Peppermint ᵀᴵ
Roman Chamomile ᵀᴵ
Wild Orange ᵀᴵ
Protocol on pg. 179

Stretch Marks

Massage 1-3 drops to affected areas 2x daily; use a carrier oil for improved efficacy.

Frankincense ᵀ
Helichrysum ᵀ
Anti-Aging Blend ᵀ
Neroli ᵀ
Yarrow ᵀ

Ailments

Stroke

Apply 2-4 drops to temples, forehead, behind ears, and back of neck 3-5x daily; ingest 2-4 drops 3x daily; diffuse several drops.

Cypress ^{A T}
Frankincense ^{A T I}
Basil ^{A T I}
Fennel ^{A T I}
Helichrysum ^{A T I}

Sunburn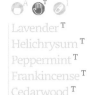

Apply 1-3 drops to affected area hourly or as needed. Blend 2-3 oils, 2-3 drops each with carrier oil for improved results.

Lavender ^T
Helichrysum ^T
Peppermint ^T
Frankincense ^T
Cedarwood ^T
Protocol on pg. 180

Teething Pain

Dilute with carrier oil and gently massage a drop along baby's jawline, reapplying as needed.

Lavender ^T
Clove ^T
Magnolia ^T
Frankincense ^T
Spikenard ^T

Tendinitis

Massage 2-4 drops into affected areas 4-5x daily, or as needed.

Lemongrass ^T
Soothing Blend ^T
Marjoram ^T
Cardamom ^T
Siberian Fir ^T

Tennis Elbow

Massage 2-4 drops into affected area as needed.

Lemongrass ^T
Soothing Blend ^T
Siberian Fir ^T
Blue Tansy ^T
Frankincense ^T

Testosterone (low)

Apply 2-4 drops to bottoms of feet and inside of thighs 2x daily; inhale from cupped hands as needed.

Patchouli ^T
Sandalwood ^T
Inspiring Blend ^T
Focus Blend ^T
Rose ^T

Thrush

Gargle 1-3 drops mixed with water several times daily; apply topically to lower throat and bottoms of feet; ingest 1-3 drops as needed.

Melaleuca ^{T I}
Geranium ^{T I}
Arborvitae ^{T I}
Oregano ^{T I}
Protective Blend ^{T I}
Protocol on pg. 180

Tick Bites

Apply 1-2 drops to bite frequently for the first hour after carefully removing tick. Dilute Oregano if necessary.

Oregano ^T
Melaleuca ^T
Cleansing Blend ^T
Lavender ^T
Outdoor Blend ^T

Tinnitus

Apply 1-2 drops behind ear 2-3x daily.

Helichrysum [T]
Grounding Blend [T]
Basil [T]
Frankincense [T]
Rosemary [T]

Tonsillitis

Gargle 1-3 drops mixed with water or ingest 3x daily; apply to outside of throat with carrier oil 3x daily.

Protective Blend [T I]
Oregano [T I]
Arborvitae [T]
Melaleuca [T I]
Melissa [T I]

Toothache

Apply a drop to gums and directly onto tooth; swish 1-3 drops with water.

Clove [T I]
Protective Blend [T I]
Helichrysum [T]
Copaiba [T I]
Wintergreen [T]

Trauma (Emotional)

Apply 2-4 drops to forehead, temples, back of neck, and chest; inhale from cupped hands as needed; diffuse several drops.

Comforting Blend [A T]
Reassuring Blend [A T]
Renewing Blend [A T]
Frankincense [A T]
Rose [A T]

Ulcers (Stomach)

Ingest 1-3 drops at least once daily; massage gently into abdomen as needed.

Lemongrass [T I]
Frankincense [T I]
Myrrh [T I]
Detoxification Blend [T I]
Geranium [T I]

Urinary Tract Infection

Massage 1-3 drops over kidneys and on bottoms of the feet; take 2-4 drops in a capsule 3x daily.

Cypress [T]
Basil [T]
Lemongrass [T I]
Juniper Berry [T I]
Cleansing Blend [T]

Varicose Veins

Massage 2-4 drops into the affected area several times daily.

Cypress [T]
Helichrysum [T]
Siberian Fir [T]
Detoxification Blend [T]
Cardamom [T]

Vision Loss

Apply 1-3 drops around eyes (do not get in eyes) and lower back 2x daily.

Clary Sage [T]
Helichrysum [T]
Anti-Aging Blend [T]
Cellular Complex [T]
Yarrow [T]

Vomiting

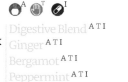

Apply 1-3 drops over stomach as needed; drink a few drops in water; inhale from cupped hands.

Digestive Blend ᴬ ᵀ ᴵ
Ginger ᴬ ᵀ ᴵ
Bergamot ᴬ ᵀ ᴵ
Peppermint ᴬ ᵀ ᴵ
Roman Chamomile ᴬ ᵀ ᴵ

Warts (common)

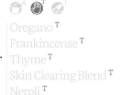

Apply a drop directly to wart several times daily until the wart disappears. Avoid the surrounding skin with Oregano.

Oregano ᵀ
Frankincense ᵀ
Thyme ᵀ
Skin Clearing Blend ᵀ
Neroli ᵀ

Wasp Sting

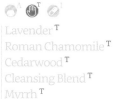

Apply one drop to sting several times daily or as needed.

Lavender ᵀ
Roman Chamomile ᵀ
Cedarwood ᵀ
Cleansing Blend ᵀ
Myrrh ᵀ

Weight Loss

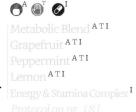

Add 2-4 drops to water to manage cravings and encourage metabolism; inhale from cupped hands to satisfy cravings.

Metabolic Blend ᴬ ᵀ ᴵ
Grapefruit ᴬ ᵀ ᴵ
Peppermint ᴬ ᵀ ᴵ
Lemon ᴬ ᵀ ᴵ
Energy & Stamina Complex ᴵ
Protocol on pg. 181

Whiplash

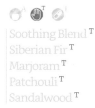

Massage 2-4 drops into affected area 2-3x daily; use with carrier oil to improve efficacy.

Soothing Blend ᵀ
Siberian Fir ᵀ
Marjoram ᵀ
Patchouli ᵀ
Sandalwood ᵀ

Withdrawal Symptoms

Apply 2-4 drops to wrists, chest, and bottoms of feet as often as needed; diffuse several drops.

Detoxification Blend ᴬ ᵀ
Cilantro ᴬ ᵀ
Cinnamon ᴬ ᵀ
Juniper Berry ᴬ ᵀ
Encouraging Blend ᴬ ᵀ

Worms

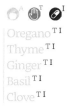

Apply 2-4 drops over abdomen, bottoms of feet, and back of neck; add 2-4 drops to water or take in capsule.

Oregano ᵀ ᴵ
Thyme ᵀ ᴵ
Ginger ᵀ ᴵ
Basil ᵀ ᴵ
Clove ᵀ ᴵ

Wrinkles

Apply 1-3 drops to affected areas as needed 2x daily; add a few drops to facial lotion or use with carrier oil for added benefits.

Anti-Aging Blend ᵀ
Frankincense ᵀ
Myrrh ᵀ
Jasmine ᵀ
Yarrow ᵀ

Section 3

Emotional Uses

Emotional Uses

The chemical constituents in oils can trigger a quick change in brain chemistry, and a fast improvement in emotions. This emotional use guide groups three related emotions, and pairs them with three oils to promote a healthier emotional state.

Use one or more of the suggested oils with these methods of application. Find what feels best for you.

Inhale from cupped hands.

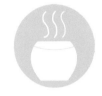

Diffuse 5-10 drops.

Wear as perfume or cologne.

Abused	Jasmine	Addicted	White Fir
Traumatized	Frankincense	Trapped	Vetiver
Abandoned	Restful Blend	Needy	Lavender
Anxious	Grounding Blend	Apathetic	Lemongrass
Panicking	Tension Blend	Disinterested	Detoxification Blend
Flustered	Neroli	Bored	Lime
Bitter	Cardamom	Confused	Roman Chamomile
Angry	Magnolia	Distracted	Focus Blend
Resentful	Siberian Fir	Purposeless	Peppermint

Emotions	Oils	Emotions	Oils
Controlled	Blue Tansy	Depressed	Joyful Blend
Powerless	Clove	Discouraged	Hopeful Blend
Shameful	Grapefruit	Disheartened	Melissa
Distressed	Tangerine	Gloomy	Uplifting Blend
Worried	Reassuring Blend	Sad	Invigorating Blend
Fearful	Black Pepper	Somber	Respiratory Blend
Grieving	Helichrysum	Insecure	Inspiring Blend
Wounded	Ylang Ylang	Unconfident	Bergamot
Hurt	Comforting Blend	Self-conscious	Coriander
Materialistic	Cilantro	Pessimistic	Bergamot
Inauthentic	Fennel	Irritable	Women's Monthly
Irresponsible	Ginger	Self-loathing	Metabolic Blend
Prideful	Cinnamon	Stubborn	Wintergreen
Jealous	Oregano	Unyielding	Juniper Berry
Controlling	Sandalwood	Inflexible	Arborvitae
Uncertain	Copaiba	Unloving	Geranium
Self-deceiving	Patchouli	Withholding	Rose
Over Stimulated	Spearmint	Unforgiving	Renewing Blend
Unmotivated	Encouraging Blend	Unsupported	Birch
Discontented	Wind Orange	Lonely	Lemon
Lethargic	Cypress	Indecisive	Cedarwood

Section 4

Single
Oils

Arborvitae
Thuja Plicata

Single Oils

Application

Chemical Constituents
a, B, y-thujaplicin
Methyl thujate
Thujic acid

Other Uses
Colds, Cold Sores, Cysts, Fevers, Intestinal Parasites, Meditation, Respiratory Viruses

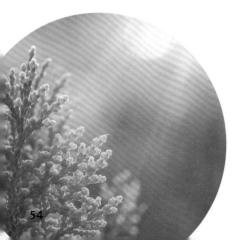

Top *Uses*

1 Strep Throat
Rub 2 drops over outside of throat, and gargle 2 drops with water.

2 Bug Repellent
Dilute with several drops of carrier oil, and rub over needed areas.

3 Skin Cancer
Apply diluted to the affected area often and in small amounts.

4 Candida
Rub 2 drops over abdomen and bladder several times a day.

5 Fungal Issues
Apply neat to needed areas.

6 Furniture Polish
Combine 4 drops with 4 drops lemon oil, and rub in using a clean rag.

Basil
Ocimum Basilicum

Application

Chemical Constituents
Linalool
Methyl chavicol
1, 8 cineol

Other Uses
Bee Stings, Bronchitis, Dizziness, Frozen Shoulder, Gout, Greasy Hair, Infertility, Lactation (increase milk supply), Loss of Sense of Smell, Migraines, Nausea, Viral Hepatitis

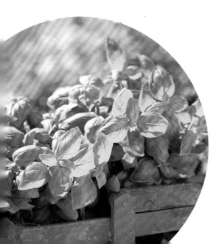

Adrenal Fatigue
Apply 1-2 drops directly to the adrenal areas or to the bottoms of the feet.

Mental Fatigue
Inhale from cupped hands, or diffuse.

Earache
Place a drop on a cotton ball, and rest over the ear for 15 minutes.

Muscle Spasms
Massage into muscles with carrier oil.

Carpal Tunnel
Massage into wrists & joints.

Cramps (abdominal)
Rub a drop clockwise over abdomen.

Cooking
Use a toothpick to add to dishes according to taste.

Bergamot
Citrus Bergamia

Application

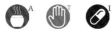

Chemical Constituents
d-limonene
Lilayl acetate
Linalol

Other Uses
Brain Injury, Colic, Depression, Fungus Issues, Irritability, Low Energy, Muscle Cramps, Oily Skin, Stress

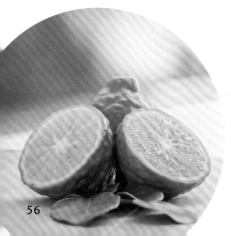

Safety
Avoid sun for 12 hours after topical application.

Top *Uses*

1 Psoriasis
Dilute 1-2 drops heavily with carrier oil, and apply frequently to affected area.

2 Sadness
Inhale from cupped hands or diffuse.

3 Appetite Loss
Drink 1-2 drops in 8 oz. water throughout the day, or diffuse.

4 Addictions
Apply to bottoms of feet, or diffuse.

5 Acne
Apply small amount to affected areas. Avoid sun for 12 hours after.

6 Self-Confidence/Self-Worth
Apply over sacral (belly button).

7 Insomnia
Use 1 drop under tongue or in water.

Black Pepper
Piper Nigrum

Application

Chemical Constituents
l-limonene
B-caryophyllene
Caryophyllene oxide

Other Uses
Antioxidant, Anxiety, Cellular Oxygenation, Diarrhea, Digestion, Gas, Emotional Repression, Inflammation, Laxative

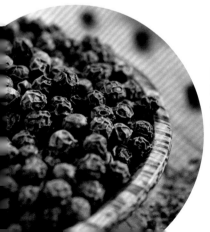

Safety
Dilute for use on sensitive skin.

1 Cold & Flu
Take 2 drops in a capsule, or apply to the bottoms of feet.

2 Smoking (quitting)
Apply to bottoms of feet (big toes) several times a day to curb cravings.

3 Circulation
Apply to bottoms of feet.

4 Sprains
Massage into muscles with carrier oil.

5 Congestion
Apply diluted over chest and upper back.

6 Airborne Viruses
Diffuse to cleanse the air.

7 Cooking
Add a drop to soups, sauces, and other dishes.

Single Oils

Blue Tansy
Tanacetum Annuum

Application

 A T I

Chemical Constituents
Sabinene
Chamazulene
Camphor

Other Uses
Bacterial Infection, Constipation, Cramping, Eczema, Fungus, Gas, Gout, Indigestion, Insect Repellent, Psoriasis, Rashes, Rheumatism, Sneezing

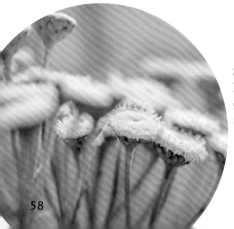

Safety
Dilute for use on sensitive skin.

Top *Uses*

1 Allergies
Put 1-2 drops under the tongue, then swallow with water after 30 seconds.

2 Arthritis & Muscle Pain
Add 5-10 drops to a bath, or massage into affected areas with carrier oil.

3 Anxiety
Apply a drop to pulse points, or diffuse.

4 Digestive Discomfort
Massage 2 drops clockwise onto stomach.

5 Dry, Itchy, or Inflamed Skin
Apply heavily diluted to affected skin.

6 Headaches
Rub a drop into temples and back of skull.

7 Congestion
Rub 2 drops onto chest and mid-back.

Cardamom
Elettaria Cardamomum

Application

 A T I

Chemical Constituents
a-terpenyl accetate
Linalol
Sabinene

Other Uses
Colitis, Constipation, Headaches, Inflammation, Menstrual Pain, Muscle Aches, Nausea, Pancreatitis, Respiratory Issues, Sore Throat, Stomach Ulcers

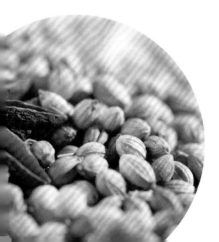

Digestive Discomfort
Drink a drop with a glass of water or in a capsule, or rub over stomach.

Congestion
Rub with carrier oil over chest, or diffuse.

Indigestion
Drink a drop with water or in a capsule.

Cough
Rub with carrier oil over chest.

Motion Sickness
Put a drop under the tongue.

Asthma, Shortness of Breath
Apply to bottoms of feet or over chest.

Cooking
Use a toothpick to add to dishes according to taste.

Cassia
Cinnamomum Cassia

Application
 A T I

Chemical Constituents
Trans-cinnamaldehyde
Eugenol
Cinnamyl accetate

Other Uses
Antiseptic, Boils, Circulation, Cold Limbs, Upset Stomach, Typhoid

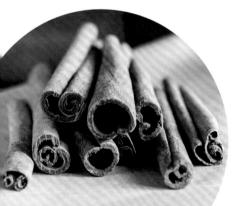

Safety
Dilute heavily for topical use. Avoid during pregnancy.

Top *Uses*

1 Vomiting
Take 1-2 drops in a capsule to restore proper digestion.

2 Viruses & Bacteria
Diffuse to cleanse the air, or take 1-2 drops in a capsule to combat internally.

3 Water Retention
Apply to bottoms of feet, take 1-2 drops in a capsule, or add 2 drops to bath.

4 Blood Sugar Balance
Take 1-2 drops in capsule with food.

5 Sex Drive
Use heavily diluted in massage, or diffuse.

6 Metabolism Boost
Apply to adrenal reflex points.

7 Cooking
Use a toothpick to add to dishes.

Cedarwood
Juniperus Virginiana

Application

Chemical Constituents
A & B-Cedrene
Trans-caryophyllene
Cedrol

Other Uses
Blemishes, Cough, Dandruff, Gums, Insect Repellent, Respiratory Function, Sinusitis, Vaginal Infection, Tension

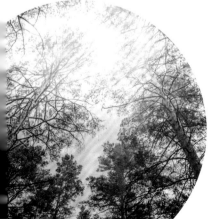

Safety
Cedarwood is very mild, and safe for even the most sensitive skin.

1 Eczema & Psoriasis
Apply neat and often to affected areas.

2 ADD/ADHD
Apply to wrists, temples, and back of neck, or diffuse.

3 Sleep
Rub onto bottoms of feet and back of neck, and diffuse. Blend with Lavender.

4 Anxiety
Apply to wrists and temples.

5 Cuts & Scrapes
Apply around wounded area to promote healing.

6 Urinary & Bladder Infection
Apply over bladder.

7 Seizures & Stroke
Apply to back of neck and bottoms of feet.

Single Oils

61

Cilantro
Coriandrum Sativum

Application

 A T I

Chemical Constituents
Tetradecanal
Cyclododecanol
Eugenol

Other Uses
Allergies, Antioxidant, Anxiety, Bloating, Gas, Liver Support, Kidney Support

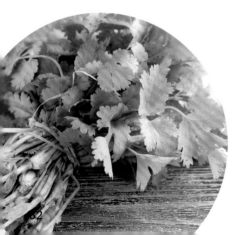

Top *Uses*

1 Heavy Metal Detox
Apply to the bottoms of feet morning and night.

2 Halitosis
Take 1-2 drops in capsule.

3 Detox
Apply over liver, kidneys, and bottoms of feet.

4 Fungal Infections
Take 1-2 drops in a capsule for internal issues, or apply topically for external issues.

5 Body Odor
Use small amounts in food, or take 1-2 drops in a capsule to deodorize internally.

6 Cooking
Use a toothpick to add to dishes according to taste.

Cinnamon
Cinnamomum Zeylanicum

Application

Chemical Constituents
Trans-cinnamaldeyde
Eugenol
Linalol

Other Uses
Airborne Bacteria, Cholesterol, Diverticulitis, Fungal Infections, General Tonic, Immune Support, Pancreas Support, Pneumonia, Typhoid, Vaginitis

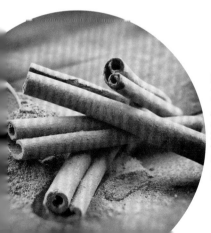

Safety
Dilute heavily. Avoid during pregnancy. Repeated use can cause sensitivity.

1. High Blood Sugar
Take 1-2 drops in capsule, or drink with large glass of water.

2. Bacterial Infection
Apply heavily diluted for external infection, or take 1-2 drops in capsule for internal infection.

3. Sex Drive
Use heavily diluted in massage, or diffuse.

4. Cavities
Swish a drop with water as a mouthwash.

5. Diabetes
Take 1-2 drops in a capsule daily.

6. Alkalinity
Drink in water to promote alkalinity.

7. Cooking
Use a toothpick to achieve desired flavor.

Single Oils

63

Clary Sage
Salvia Sclarea

Application

 A T I

Chemical Constituents
Linalyl acetate
Linalol
Sclareol

Other Uses
Aneurysm, Breast Enlargement, Cholesterol, Convulsions, Endometriosis, Epilepsy, Fragile Hair, Hot Flashes, Impotence, Lactation, Parkinson's, Premenopause, Seizure

Safety
Use with caution during pregnancy.

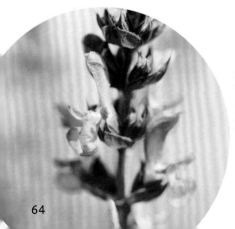

Top *Uses*

1 Hormone Balance
Apply to wrists and behind ears.

2 PMS
Apply to bottoms of feet, or take 1-2 drops in capsule.

3 Postpartum Depression
Diffuse or apply over heart area.

4 Abdominal Cramps
Massage over abdomen.

5 Pink Eye
Apply carefully around edge of eye.

6 Infertility
Apply to abdomen & uterine reflex points, or take 1-2 drops in capsule.

7 Breast Cancer
Apply diluted to breasts, or take 1-2 drops in capsule to regulate estrogen levels.

Clove
Eugenia Caryophyllata

Application
A T I

Chemical Constituents
Eugenol
Eugenyl Acetate
B-caryophyllene

Other Uses
Addictions, Blood Clots, Candida, Cataracts, Fever, Herpes Simplex, Hodgkin's Disease, Glaucoma, Gingivitis, Lipoma, Lupus, Lyme Disease, Macular Degeneration, Memory Loss, Parasites, Termites

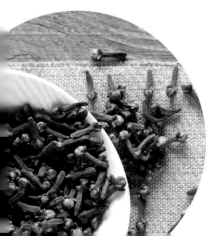

Safety
Can irritate sensitive skin. Use with caution during pregnancy.

Top *Uses*

1 Thyroid (hypo, Hashimoto's)
Apply diluted over thyroid or to thyroid reflex point, or take 1-2 drops in capsule.

2 Toothache
Apply directly to problematic tooth.

3 Smoking Addiction
Rub onto bottom of big toe.

4 Immune Support
Take 1-2 drops in a capsule.

5 Antioxidant
Take 1-2 drops in a capsule, or use in cooking.

6 Liver Detox
Rub over liver or on liver reflex point.

7 Rheumatoid Arthritis
Massage diluted into affected area.

Single Oils

65

Copaiba
Copaifera Officinalis

Application

Chemical Constituents
d-Limonene
y-terpinene
Lilayl acetate

Other Uses
Anxiety, Congestion, Infection, Mood Disorders, Nail Fungus, Skin Strengthening

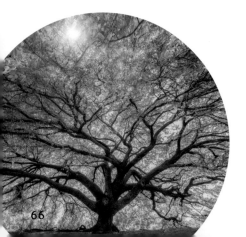

Top *Uses*

1 Headache & Migraine
Massage gently onto temples, scalp, and the back of the neck.

2 Pain & Inflammation
Inhale or diffuse, or apply topically to affected areas.

3 Wrinkles, Pimples, Blisters
Apply daily with a carrier oil.

4 High Blood Pressure
Apply to the bottoms of feet twice daily.

5 Athlete's Foot
Apply several drops to clean, dry feet.

6 Detox
Apply over bladder to stimulate detox through urination.

Coriander
Coriandrum Sativum

Application
 A T I

Chemical Constituents
Linalol
a-pinene
Geranyl

Other Uses
Alzheimer's, Itchy Skin, Joint Pain, Low Energy, Measles, Muscle Tone, Muscle Spasms, Nausea, Neuropathy, Stiffness, Whiplash

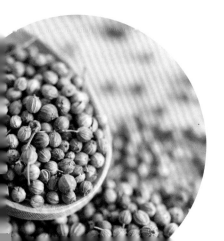

Top *Uses*

1 Diabetes (high blood sugar)
Combine with 1 drop Cinnamon & Juniper Berry in capsule daily.

2 Food Poisoning
Drink 2 drops in water, or take in capsule.

3 Body Odor
Drink 2 drops in water, or take in capsule.

4 Cartilage Injury
Massage into affected area with carrier oil.

5 Rashes
Apply diluted to affected area.

6 Muscle Aches
Take a drop in a capsule, or massage with carrier oil onto affected muscles.

7 Cooking
Use a toothpick to add desired flavor.

Cypress
Cupressus Sempervirens

Application

Chemical Constituents
a-pinene
Cedrol
a-terpinyl acetate

Other Uses
Aneurysm, Bunions, Edema, Hemorrhoids, Flu, Incontinence, Lou Gehrig's Disease, Ovary Issues, Prostate Issues, Raynaud's Disease, Tuberculosis, Varicose Veins, Whooping Cough

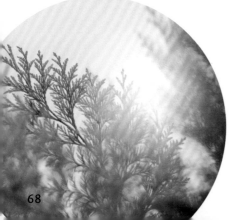

Safety
Can irritate sensitive skin. Use with caution during pregnancy.

Top *Uses*

1 Circulation (poor)
Apply 2 drops to the bottoms of each foot morning and night.

2 Bladder/Urinary Tract Infection
Massage 2 drops with carrier oil over bladder. Repeat every 2 hours as needed.

3 Bone Spurs
Apply directly onto affected area.

4 Concussion
Massage 2 drops with carrier oil into back of neck, back of skull, and shoulders.

5 Restless Leg Syndrome
Massage 2 drops with carrier oil into bottoms of feet, calves, and upper legs.

6 Bed Wetting
Apply 2 drops neat over bladder before bed.

Single Oils

68

Douglas Fir
Pseudotsuga Menziesil

Application

 A T I

Chemical Constituents
Linalol
a-pinene
Geranyl

Other Uses
Arthritis, Constipation, Depression, Emotional Congestion, Energy, Generational Patterns, Weight Gain, Sinus Issues

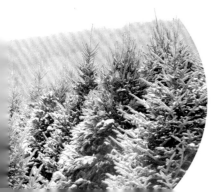

Top *Uses*

1 Muscle Soreness
Rub 2-4 drops with carrier oil onto sore muscles.

2 Congestion
Rub 1-2 drops over chest, or diffuse.

3 Headache & Migraine
Rub a drop into temples.

4 Focus & Mental Clarity
Inhale from cupped hands, or diffuse.

5 Skin Irritations
Apply heavily diluted to irritated skin.

6 Household Cleansing
Use with Lemon oil for a refreshing household cleaner.

7 Cough
Apply 1-2 drops to chest or lung reflex points.

Eucalyptus
Eucalyptus Radiata

Application

Chemical Constituents
1,8 ceneol
a & B-pinenes
a-terpineol

Other Uses
Colds, Fever, Flu, Headache, Earaches, Insect Bites & Stings, Kidney Stones, Muscle Aches, Neuralgia, Rheumatism, Rhinitis

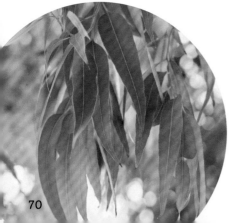

Safety
Not for use topically on newborns.

Top *Uses*

1 Congestion & Cough
Apply 2-4 drops to chest, or diffuse.

2 Bronchitis & Pneumonia
Apply 2-4 drops to chest & mid-back, or diffuse.

3 Sinusitis
Apply heavily diluted to sinuses, carefully avoiding eyes.

4 Asthma
Inhale 2 drops from cupped hands, and apply to lung reflex points.

5 Menstrual Cramp
Rub 1-2 drops with carrier oil over abdomen.

6 Mental Fatigue
Inhale 1-2 drops from cupped hands, or diffuse.

Fennel
Foeniculum Vulgare

Application

Chemical Constituents
Trans-anethole
Trans-ocimene
Linalol

Other Uses
Blood Sugar Imbalance, Constipation, Digestive Disorders, Edema, Fertility Issues, Fluid Retention, Intestinal Parasites, Menopause, PMS, Spasms, Stroke

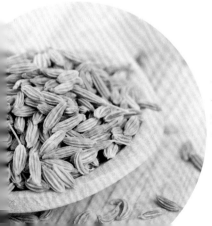

Safety
Use with caution if pregnant. Avoid if epileptic.

Top Uses

1 Flatulence
Rub 1-2 drops over outside of stomach, or drink with water.

2 Milk Supply (low)
Massage 1 drop diluted around nipples 2-3 times daily.

3 Digestive Disorders
Drink 1-2 drops in water or capsule.

4 Nausea
Rub 1-2 drops over stomach, or drink a drop in water.

5 Menstrual Discomfort
Rub a drop over abdomen.

6 Parasites
Drink 2-4 drops in a capsule.

7 Colic
Rub a drop diluted over stomach.

Frankincense
Boswellia Frereana

Application

A T I

Chemical Constituents
a-phellandrenes
B-elemene
Cis-verbenol

Other Uses
ADHD, Aneurysm, Asthma, Balance, Brain Health, Coma, Concussion, Fibroids, Genital Warts, Immune Support, Lou Gehrig's Disease, Memory, Moles, MRSA, Multiple Sclerosis, Scarring, Sciatica, Warts, Wrinkles

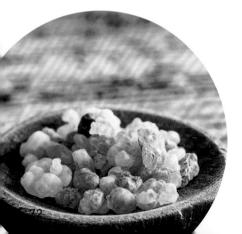

Top *Uses*

1 Depression & Anxiety
Use a drop under the tongue, apply to pulse points, or diffuse.

2 Alzheimer's & Dementia
Apply 2 drops to bottoms of feet and base of skull twice daily.

3 Cellular Function
Take 1-2 drops in capsule.

4 Pain & Inflammation
Use a drop under the tongue, or massage into inflamed areas.

5 Parkinson's
Apply 1-2 drops to brain reflex points, and diffuse.

6 Cancer
Take 1-2 drops in capsule, and apply close to the affected area frequently.

Geranium
Pelargonium Graveolens

Application

Chemical Constituents
Citronellol
Citronellyl Formate
Isomenthone

Other Uses
Bleeding, Circulation, Depression, Diarrhea, Gastric Ulcers, Hernia, Low Libido, Menstrual Cramps, Menopause, Neuralgia, Raynaud's Disease, Spasms, Vertigo

Safety
Possible skin sensitivity.

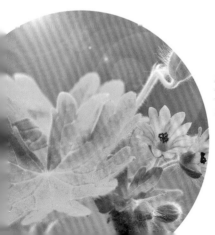

Top *Uses*

1 Liver & Kidney Support
Rub a drop directly over liver and kidneys.

2 Autism
Apply 1-2 drops to bottoms of feet, or diffuse.

3 Jaundice
Apply 1 drop diluted to bottoms of feet, and diffuse.

4 PMS & Hormone Balance
Apply a drop to pulse points.

5 Hemorrhoids
Apply heavily diluted to affected areas.

6 Reproductive Disorders (female)
Apply 1-2 drops to reproductive reflex points.

7 Varicose Veins
Massage diluted into affected areas.

Ginger
Zingiber Officinale

Application

Chemical Constituents
Zingiberene
Camphene
Nonanol

Other Uses
Aneurysm, Breast Enlargement, Cholesterol, Convulsions, Endometriosis, Epilepsy, Fragile Hair, Hot Flashes, Impotence, Lactation, Parkinson's, Premenopause, Seizure

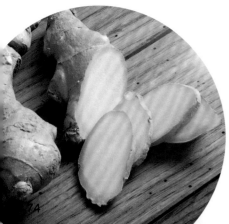

Safety
Possible skin sensitivity.

Top *Uses*

1 Nausea & Stomach Upset
Drink 1-2 drops in capsule.

2 Vomiting
Rub a drop heavily diluted over stomach.

3 Constipation
Apply 1-2 drops diluted over stomach, or take in capsule.

4 Immune Support
Apply 1-2 drops to bottoms of feet, or drink in capsule.

5 Congestion & Cough
Diffuse 3-6 drops.

6 Cold & Flu
Apply 1-2 drops to bottoms of feet, or drink in capsule.

7 Cooking
Use toothpick to achieve desired taste.

Grapefruit
Citrus X Paradisi

Application

 A T I

Chemical Constituents
d-Limonene
Nonanal
Nootketone

Other Uses
Anorexia, Bulimia, Dry Throat, Edema, Energy, Hangovers, Jet Lag, Lymphatic Congestion, Miscarriage Recovery, Obesity, Overeating

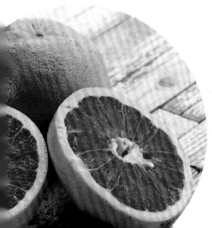

Safety
Avoid sun exposure for 12 hours after topical use.

1 Detox
Drink 1-3 drops in water.

2 Weight Loss
Apply 10 drops diluted with carrier oil over cellulite and fatty areas.

3 Smoking Addiction
Drink 1-3 drops in water after meals.

4 Antiviral Support
Apply 1-2 drops to bottoms of feet, or drink in water.

5 Appetite Suppressant
Diffuse several drops, or drink in water.

6 Gallbladder Stones
Drink 1-3 drops in water 3 times daily.

7 Food & Cooking
Use in smoothies, dressings, and sauces.

Single Oils

Green Mandarin
Citrus Nobilis

Application

Chemical Constituents
d-limonene
y-terpinene
linalool, myrcene

Other Uses
Antibacterial, Anti-viral, Depression, Numbness, Regenerative, Skin Toner

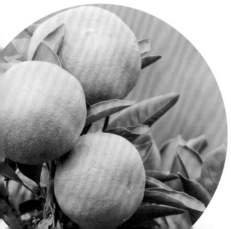

Safety
Excessive dosing may cause indigestion. Does not cause photosensitivity.

Top *Uses*

1 Nerve Damage
Apply 2-4 drops to bottoms of feet and along spine.

2 Sensation Loss in Extremities
Massage with carrier oil into affected areas.

3 Pain
Massage 2 drops into affected areas.

4 Simple Antibiotic
Take 2-4 drops in a capsule 3-5x daily as needed.

5 Mood Lift
Diffuse 3-6 drops or inhale from cupped hands as needed.

6 Ageless Skin
Apply 2 drops with carrier oil to fine lines and wrinkles before bed.

Helichrysum
Helichrysum Italicum

Application
 A T I

Chemical Constituents
Neryl Acetate
Italidione
y-curcumene

Other Uses
AIDS/HIV, Broken Blood Vessels, Bruises, Cuts, Earache, Fibroids, Gallbladder Infection, Hemorrhaging, Hernias, Herpes, Lymphatic Drainage, Nose Bleed, Sciatica, Staph Infection, Stretch Marks, Wrinkles

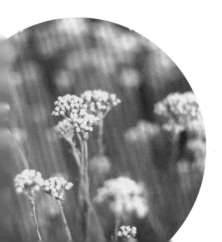

Top *Uses*

1 Tissue Repair
Apply neat or diluted to wounds.

2 Bleeding
Apply to clean wound to stop bleeding.

3 Eczema & Psoriasis
Apply 1-2 drops diluted to affected areas.

4 Shock
Diffuse 3-6 drops.

5 Tinnitus
Apply a drop behind ear.

6 Viral Infections
Take 1-2 drops in capsule, or diffuse.

7 Cholesterol
Take 1-3 drops in capsule, and apply to bottoms of feet.

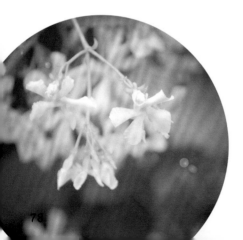

Jasmine
Jasminum Grandiflorum

Application

A T I

Chemical Constituents
Benzyl Acetate
Phytol
Squalene

Other Uses
Apathy, Anxiety, Dry Skin, Insecurity, Labor & Delivery, Low Libido, Menstrual Camps, Nervous Tension, Nervousness, Ovulation, Stress

Top *Uses*

1 Depression & Self-Esteem Issues
Inhale 1-2 drops from cupped hands, or apply over heart.

2 Wrinkles & Fine Lines
Apply directly to desired areas.

3 Pink Eye
Apply carefully around affected eye, avoiding the eye itself.

4 Infertility
Apply to pulse points and reproductive reflex points.

5 Cramps & Spasms
Apply 1-2 drops to needed areas.

6 Lethargy & Fatigue
Inhale from cupped hands, or diffuse.

7 Sleep & Relaxation
Apply to bottoms of feet and temples.

Juniper Berry
Juniperus Communis

Application

Chemical Constituents
a-pinene
B-caryophyllene
Bornyl Acetate

Other Uses
Acne, Anxiety, Bacteria, Bloating, Cellulite, Cystitis, Detoxifying, Fluid Retention, Heavy Legs, Jaundice, Menstrual Cramps, Mental Exhaustion, Stress, Ulcers, Viruses

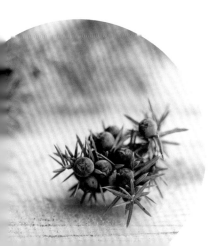

Top *Uses*

1 Kidney Detox & Infections
Rub 1-2 drops over kidneys, or take in capsule.

2 Diabetes
Take 1-2 drops in capsule daily.

3 Kidney Stones
Apply 1-2 drops over kidneys.

4 Urinary Tract Infection
Apply 1-2 drops over bladder.

5 High Cholesterol
Take 1-2 drops in capsule, or apply to bottoms of feet.

6 Tinnitus
Apply a drop behind affected ear.

7 Chronic Fatigue
Apply 1-2 drops to pulse points, or diffuse.

Lavender
Lavandula Angustifolia

Application

 A T I

Chemical Constituents

Linalol
Linalyl Acetate
B-ocimene

Other Uses

Allergies, Bites, Blisters, Chicken Pox, Club Foot, Colic, Convulsions, Crying, Dandruff, Diaper Rash, Gangrene, Giardia, Impetigo, Insomnia, Poison Ivy & Oak, Seizures, Stings, Tachycardia, Teething Pain, Ticks

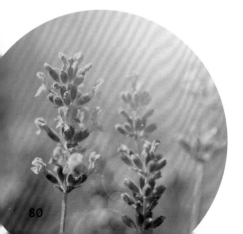

Top *Uses*

1 Stress & Anxiety
Apply 1-2 drops to temples, or diffuse.

2 Sleep
Apply 2 drops to bottoms of feet and temples, or diffuse near bedside.

3 Skin Irritations & Burns
Apply 1-2 drops with carrier oil.

4 Allergies & Hay Fever
Put a drop under tongue for 30 seconds, then swallow with water.

5 Cuts, Blisters, & Scrapes
Apply diluted to affected areas.

6 Irritability
Apply 1-2 drops to pulse points.

7 Headaches & Migraines
Apply 1-2 drops to temples and base of skull.

Lemon
Citrus Limon

Application

Chemical Constituents
d-Limonene
Citral
Hexanol

Other Uses
Anxiety, Cold Sores, Colds, Concentration, Constipation, Depression, Disinfectant, Dysentery, Flu, Furniture Polish, Greasy Hair, High Blood Pressure, Kidney Stones, MRSA, Pancreatitis, Parasites, Tonsillitis

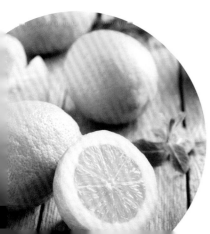

Safety
Avoid sun exposure for 12 hours after topical use.

Top Uses

1 Energy
Inhale 1-2 drops from cupped hands.

2 Detox
Drink 1-3 drops in water, or apply to bottoms of feet.

3 Permanent Marker
Rub several drops with clean rag.

4 Sore Throat
Take 1-2 drops with a spoonful of honey.

5 Increase Alkalinity
Drink 1-3 drops in water.

6 Household Cleaner
Use several drops with water in glass spray bottle.

7 Food & Cooking
Use in smoothies, juices, and sauces.

Single Oils

Lemongrass
Cymbopogon Flexuosus

Application

 A T I

Chemical Constituents
Geranial
a-terpineol
Farnesol

Other Uses
Airborne Bacteria, Bladder Infection, Carpal Tunnel, Charley Horses, Connective Tissue Injury, Constipation, Frozen Shoulder, Lymphatic Drainage, Paralysis, Sprains, Urinary Tract Infection

Single Oils

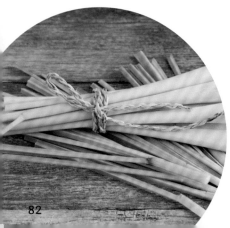

Safety
Possible skin sensitivity. Do not use internally more than 10 days in a row.

Top *Uses*

1 Thyroid Support (hypo & hyper)
Apply a drop diluted over thyroid.

2 High Cholesterol
Take 1-2 drops in capsule.

3 Ligament & Tendon Issues
Apply 1-2 drops diluted to painful areas.

4 Stomach Ulcers
Take 1 drop in capsule.

5 Immune Support
Apply 1-2 drops to bottoms of feet.

6 Lactose Intolerance
Take 1 drop in capsule.

7 Cooking
Use toothpick to achieve desired flavor.

Lime
Citrus Aurantifolia

Application

A T I

Chemical Constituents
d-Limonene
1,8 cineol
Geranial

Other Uses
Antiviral Support, Blood Pressure, Cellulite, Depression, Detox, Energy, Exhaustion, Fever, Gallstones, Gum Removal, Herpes, Memory, Water Purification

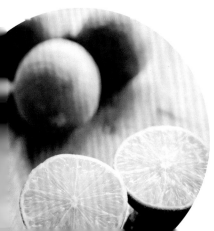

Safety
Avoid sun exposure for 12 hours after topical use.

1 Chronic Cough
Apply 2-4 drops over chest, mid-back, and lung reflex points.

2 Colds
Drink 1-3 drops in water, and diffuse.

3 Sore Throat
Gargle 2 drops with water.

4 Cold Sores
Apply 1 drop diluted to affected area.

5 Antioxidant
Drink 1-3 drops in water.

6 Bacterial Infections
Apply 1-2 drops with carrier oil to affected area.

7 Mental Clarity
Diffuse 3-6 drops, or inhale from cupped hands.

Single Oils

Litsea
Litsea Cubeba

Application

Chemical Constituents
Geranial
Neral
Limonene

Other Uses
Anxiety, Cold, Cough, Disinfectant, Household Cleaning, Insect Repellent, Odors, Perspiration, Sleep, Stress

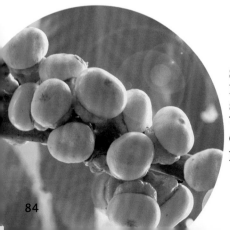

Safety
Possible skin sensitivity. Use with caution during pregnancy.

Top *Uses*

1 Emotional Balance
Diffuse several drops, or wear on scarf or sleeve throughout the day.

2 Mental Rejuvenation
Inhale 1-2 drops from cupped hands.

3 Postpartum Depression
Diffuse, or apply over heart area.

4 E. Coli
Apply 1-2 drops diluted to affected areas.

5 Internal Bacterial Infections
Drink 2-4 drops in water or in a capsule.

6 Aging
Apply 1-2 drops in facial lotion to combat age-promoting free radicals.

7 Athlete's Foot
Apply 1-2 drops to clean feet.

Magnolia
Michelia X Alba

Application

Chemical Constituents
Linalool
β-caryophyllene
Selinene
(E)-B-Ocimene

Other Uses
Anger Issues, Bronchitis, Excess Mucus, Heart Health, Motion Sickness, Nervous System Support

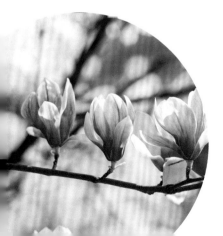

Top *Uses*

1 Stress & Anxiety
Apply to wrists and temples, taking deep breaths.

2 Menstrual Cramping
Apply over lower abdomen and to wrists.

3 Sore Muscles
Massage onto affected muscles with carrier oil.

4 Depression
Apply over heart in the morning and afternoon.

5 Hives & Rashes
Apply with carrier oil to affected skin.

6 Cough
Apply over chest and mid-back.

7 Chronic Pain
Diffuse 3-6 drops or apply to wrists, spine, and bottoms of feet.

Manuka
Leptospermum Scoparium

Application

Chemical Constituents
Eugenol
Eugenyl Acetate
B-caryophyllene

Other Uses
Athlete's Foot, Bronchitis, Catarrh, Contusions, Cough, Fungal Skin Infections, Head Lice, Influenza, Scabies, Skin Infection, Ulceration

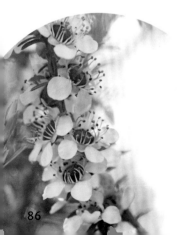

Safety
Possible skin sensitivity. Use with caution when pregnant.

Top *Uses*

1 Blemishes & Complexion
Add a couple drops to skincare products, or apply diluted to affected areas.

2 Hypertension
Apply 1-2 drops to pulse points, or diffuse.

3 Air Purification
Diffuse 4-8 drops.

4 Sleep
Graze pillows with a drop of oil, and diffuse near bedside.

5 Bronchial Infection
Inhale 1-2 drops from cupped hands, or diffuse.

6 Ringworm & Parasites
Apply 1-2 drops diluted to affected areas.

Marjoram
Origanum Majorana

Application

Chemical Constituents
a & y-terpinenes
a-terpineol
terpinen-4-ol

Other Uses
Arterial Vasodilator, Bruises, Colic, Constipation, Croup, Headache, Gastrointestinal Disorders, Insomnia, Menstrual Problems, Parkinson's, Prolapsed Mitral Valve, Ringworm, Sprains, Whiplash

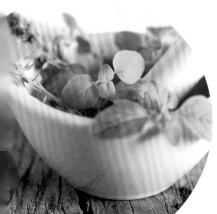

Safety
Use with caution during pregnancy.

Top *Uses*

1 Muscle Injury
Massage 2 drops with carrier oil into injured muscles.

2 Carpal Tunnel & Arthritis
Apply 1-2 drops neat to affected area.

3 High Blood Pressure
Apply 2 drops to bottoms of feet, or take in a capsule.

4 Irritable Bowel Syndrome
Take 1-2 drops in a capsule, or rub over abdomen.

5 Diverticulitis
Take 1-2 drops in a capsule.

6 Pancreatitis
Apply 1-2 drops neat over pancreas area.

7 Chronic Stress
Rub 1-2 drops onto back of neck.

Single Oils

87

Melaleuca
Melaleuca Alternifolia

Application

Chemical Constituents
a- & y-terpinenes
Terpinen-4-ol
a- & o-cadinenes

Other Uses
Aneurysm, Bacterial Infections, Cankers, Candida, Cavities, Cold Sores, Cuts, Dermatitis, Ear Infections, Fungal Infections, Hepatitis, Infected Wounds, MRSA, Nail Fungus, Pink Eye, Rubella, Thrush

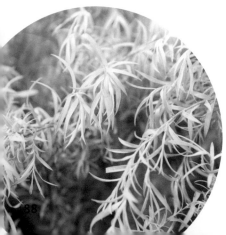

Safety
Possible skin sensitivity.

Top *Uses*

1 Rashes & Eczema
Apply 1-2 drops diluted to affected areas.

2 Dandruff
Add 2 drops to shampoo daily.

3 Athlete's Foot
Apply 1-2 drops neat to clean feet.

4 Acne & Blemishes
Apply a dab to affected areas.

5 Staph Infections
Take 1-2 drops in capsule.

6 Strep Throat & Tonsillitis
Gargle 2 drops with water, and rub 1-2 drops diluted to outside of throat.

7 Herpes
Apply 1 drop diluted to affected areas.

Melissa
Melissa Officinalis

Application
 A T I

Chemical Constituents
Geranial
Germacrene-D
Linalol

Other Uses
Allergies, Anxiety, Blisters, Colds, Dysentery, Erysipelas, Hypertension, Nervousness, Sleep Disorders, Sterility, Viral Outbreak

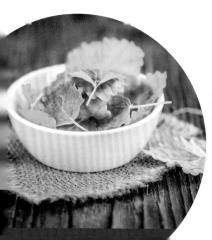

Safety
Dilute for sensitive skin.

1 Viral Infections
Take 1-2 drops in a capsule.

2 Cold Sores & Herpes
Apply a drop to affected areas.

3 Depression
Use thumb to hold a drop to the roof of the mouth.

4 Bronchitis, Asthma
Apply 1-2 drops diluted over chest.

5 Neurotonic
Apply a drop to the bottoms of feet.

6 Shock
Apply a drop diluted to back of neck, or diffuse.

7 Insomnia
Apply a drop to big toe, or use thumb to hold a drop to the roof of mouth.

Single Oils

Myrrh
Commiphora Myrrha

Application
 A T I

Chemical Constituents
Lindestrene
Methoxyfurogermacrene
Curzenone

Other Uses
Cancer, Chapped Skin, Congestion, Dysentery, Gum Bleeding, Hepatitis, Liver Cirrhosis, Scabies, Stretch Marks

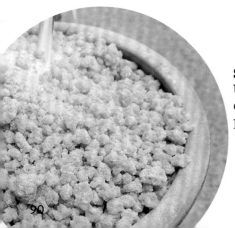

Top *Uses*

1 Wrinkles & Fine Lines
Massage into needed areas as desired.

2 Gum Disease & Issues
Apply 1-2 drops to gums, or swish with water as mouth rinse.

3 Thyroid Support
Rub 1-2 drops over thyroid.

4 Anxiety & Depression
Inhale 1-2 drops from cupped hands, or diffuse.

5 Mucus & Bronchitis
Apply 1-2 drops to chest, or diffuse.

6 Eczema & Skin Infections
Apply 1-2 drops to affected areas.

7 Nail Fungus
Apply a drop to affected nails.

Safety
Use with caution during pregnancy.

Neroli
Citrus Aurantium

Application

Chemical Constituents
Linalool
Geraniol
Limonene

Other Uses
Convalescence, Indigestion, Insomnia, Intestinal Cramping, Menopausal Anxiety, Sleep Disorders, Tension

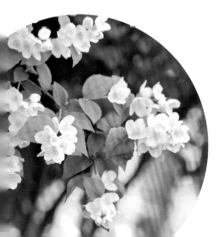

Top *Uses*

1 Scar Tissue & Stretch Marks
Massage a few drops with carrier oil into needed areas.

2 Perfume
Apply 1-2 drops to pulse points.

3 Cramps & Spasms
Apply neat to affected areas.

4 Emotional Exhaustion
Inhale from cupped hands, or diffuse.

5 Nervousness
Apply a drop to pulse points.

6 Depression
Wear as perfume, inhale from cupped hands, or diffuse.

7 Skin Regeneration
Apply generously to damaged or worn skin.

Oregano
Origanum Vulgare

Application

Chemical Constituents
Carvacrol
B-caryophyllene
Rosmaric Acid

Other Uses
Athlete's Foot, Calluses, Canker Sores, Carpal Tunnel, Control Issues, Ebola, Fungal Infections, Intestinal Parasites, MRSA, Nasal Polyps, Plague, Ringworm

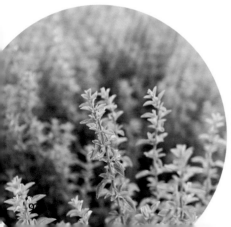

Safety
Heavily dilute for topical use. Do not use internally for more than 10 days in a row.

Top *Uses*

1 Bacterial & Viral Infection
Take 1-3 drops in a capsule for internal issues.

2 Warts
Apply directly to wart with toothpick, avoiding surrounding skin.

3 Candida & Staph Infection
Take 1-3 drops in a capsule.

4 Pneumonia & Whooping Cough
Diffuse 1-3 drops, sitting nearby the diffuser for several minutes. Also rub onto bottoms of feet.

5 Rheumatoid Arthritis
Massage 1 drop heavily diluted into affected area. Also take in a capsule.

6 Strep Throat & Tonsillitis
Gargle a drop in water. Also take 1-3 drops in capsule.

Patchouli
Pogostemon Cablin

Application

Chemical Constituents
a-bulesene
Patchoulol
Pathoulenone

Other Uses
Abscess, Cellulite, Chapped Skin, Depression, Dermatitis, Hemorrhoids, Hives, Irritability, Mastitis, Parasitic Skin Infection, PMS, Weeping Wounds

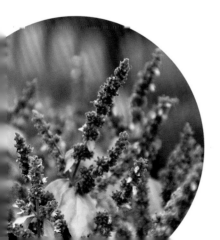

1 Diuretic
Apply 1-2 drops over lower abdomen.

2 Wrinkle Prevention
Add a drop to toner or moisturizer.

3 Shingles
Take 1-2 drops in capsule, or apply to bottoms of feet.

4 Dopamine Shortage
Diffuse 2-4 drops, or apply to pulse points.

5 Dandruff
Massage 1-2 drops into clean, dry scalp after showering.

6 Weight Loss
Take 1-2 drops with other weight loss essential oils in a capsule.

Single Oils

Peppermint
Menta Piperita

Application
 A T I

Chemical Constituents
Menthol
a & B-pinenes
Germacrene-D

Other Uses
Alertness, Allergies, Autism, Burns, Cravings, Gastritis, Hangover, Hot Flashes, Hypothyroidism, Loss of Sense of Smell, Memory, Milk Supply (Decrease), Osteoporosis, Sciatica, Sinusitis, Typhoid

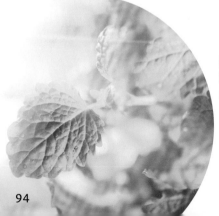

Safety
Possible skin sensitivity.

Top *Uses*

1 Headache & Migraine
Massage 1-2 drops into temples and base of skull, avoiding the eyes.

2 Digestive Upset
Drink 1-2 drops in water, or massage directly over stomach.

3 Asthma & Cough
Apply 2 drops with carrier oil over chest and lung reflex points, or diffuse.

4 Bad Breath
Lick a dab from your finger.

5 Low Energy & Mental Fog
Drink 1-2 drops in water, or diffuse.

6 Muscle & Joint Pain
Rub a drop diluted into affected areas.

7 Fevers
Apply 1-2 drops to back of neck.

Petitgrain
Citrus Aurantium

Application

Chemical Constituents
Linalyl acetate
Linalool
Alpha-terpineol

Other Uses
Abdominal Cramps/Spasms, Aches, Acne, Convalescence, Depression, Hysteria, Infected Wounds, Nausea, Nervous Asthma, Oily Hair, Shock, Stress-Related Conditions, Tension

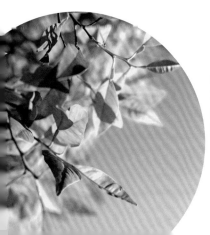

Safety
Use with caution during pregnancy.

Top Uses

1 Nervous & Muscular Spasms
Apply 1-2 drops to bottoms of feet, or to area of spasm.

2 Seizures
Apply 1-2 drops to bottoms of feet and back of neck.

3 Insomnia
Use a drop under tongue, or on pulse points. Also diffuse.

4 Irritability & Stress
Apply a drop behind ears, or wear as cologne on pulse points.

5 Bacterial Infections
Apply topically to affected area, or take 1-3 drops in a capsule.

6 Spastic Coughing
Apply 1-2 drops with carrier oil over chest and mid-back, or diffuse.

Pink Pepper
Schinus Molle

Application

 A T I

Chemical Constituents
B-Myrcene, a-Phellandrene, p-Cymene, d-Cadinene, Limonene, B-Phellandrene

Other Uses
Arthritis, Bee Stings, Cancer, Chest Pain, Colds, Emotional Upset, Flu, Seizures

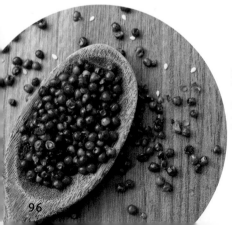

Safety
Use with caution during pregnancy.

Top *Uses*

1 Cancer Prevention
Take 2-4 drops in a veggie capsule or massage with carrier oil 2x daily.

2 Muscle Spasms
Massage 2-3 drops with carrier oil into affected areas.

3 Circulatory Disorders
Massage 2 drops with carrier oil into legs.

4 Pain Relief
Take 2 drops in a capsule as needed.

5 Convulsions
Use 2-4 drops on the bottoms of feet, or take 5 drops in a capsule.

6 High Blood Pressure
Apply 3 drops with a carrier oil to chest.

7 Cough Suppressant
Apply 5 drops with carrier oil to chest and upper back.

Roman Chamomile
Anthemis Nobilis

Application

Chemical Constituents
Isobutyl
a- & B-pinenes
Pinocarvone

Other Uses
Allergies, Anorexia, Bee/Hornet Stings, Club Foot, Dysentery, Hyperactivity, Menopause, Muscle Spasms, Neuralgia, Rashes, Shock, Sore Nipples

Top *Uses*

1 Sleep & Insomnia
Apply 1-2 drops to temples and wrists, or diffuse next to bedside.

2 Panic Attacks
Carry on person and breathe a drop deeply from cupped hands as needed.

3 Diaper Rash
Apply 1 drop heavily diluted with carrier oil to baby skin.

4 Crying
Add a drop to front of shirt or sleeve, or diffuse.

5 PMS & Cramps
Apply a drop over abdomen.

6 Parasites & Worms
Apply 1-2 drops over abdomen, and take in a capsule.

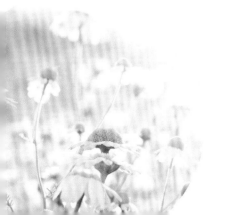

Rose
Rosa Damascena

Application

Chemical Constituents
Citronellol
Stearoptene
Nonadecane

Other Uses
Anxiety, Astringent, Dysmenorrhea, Endometriosis, Grief, Facial Redness, Impotency, Infertility, Irregular Ovulation, Menstrual Cramping, Phobias

Safety
Use with caution during pregnancy.

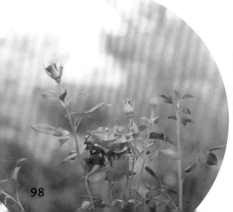

1 Aging Skin
Add a drop to toner or moisturizer, or apply with carrier oil over fine lines, wrinkles, and age spots.

2 Low Libido
Apply 1-2 drops to pulse points, or to reproductive reflex points.

3 Scar Tissue
Massage into scar tissue 3 times daily.

4 Self-Esteem & Depression
Apply 1-2 drops over heart, or diffuse.

5 Aphrodisiac
Diffuse a few drops, or wear on pulse points.

6 Poison Ivy/Oak
Apply 1-2 drops diluted to irritated areas.

Rosemary
Rosmarinus Officinalis

Application
A T I

Chemical Constituents
1, 8 Cineol
a-pinene
Camphor

Other Uses
Alcohol Addiction, Adenitis, Arthritis, Bell's Palsy, Cellulite, Club Foot, Constipation, Headaches, Kidney Infection, Lice, Muscular Dystrophy, Osteoarthritis, Schmidt's Syndrome, Sinusitis

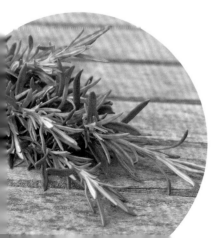

Safety
Avoid during pregnancy, if epileptic, or with high blood pressure.

1. Chronic Cough
Apply 2-4 drops to lung reflex points or diluted over chest, or diffuse.

2. Mental & Adrenal Fatigue
Inhale 1-2 drops from cupped hands, or take in a capsule.

3. Focus & Memory Issues
Apply a drop over forehead, or diffuse.

4. Cold & Flu
Apply 1-2 drops diluted over chest.

5. Low Blood Pressure
Massage with carrier oil into legs and on bottoms of feet.

6. Jet Lag
Apply 1-2 drops to temples after flying.

7. Hair Loss.
Work 2 drops into scalp before washing.

Single Oils

Sandalwood
Santalum Album

Single Oils

Application

Chemical Constituents
a & B-santalols
a- & B-santalenes
Norticycloekasantalic Acid

Other Uses
Aphrodisiac, Back Pain, Blemishes, Calming, Cartilage Repair, Coma, Dry Skin/Scalp, Exhaustion, Hiccups, Laryngitis, Lou Gehrig's Disease, Moles, Multiple Sclerosis, UV Radiation, Yoga

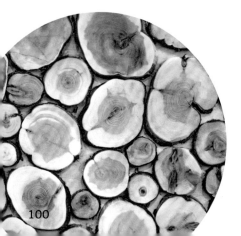

100

Top *Uses*

1 Rashes & Skin Conditions
Apply 1-2 drops with carrier oil to affected areas.

2 Cancer & Tumors
Take 1-2 drops in capsule, apply diluted to affected area, or diffuse.

3 Meditation
Apply a drop to temples during meditation.

4 Low Testosterone
Take 1-2 drops in a capsule, or apply to pulse points and lower abdomen.

5 Scars
Massage 1-2 drops into scars often.

6 Alzheimer's Disease
Apply 1-2 drops to base of skull, or take 1-2 drops in capsule daily.

Siberian Fir
Abies Sibirica

Application

Chemical Constituents
Bornyl Acetate
Terpinyl Acetate
Camphene

Other Uses
Anxiety, Bronchitis, Catarrh, Fever, Sinus-
itis, Sluggish Nerves, Tension, Urinary
Infection

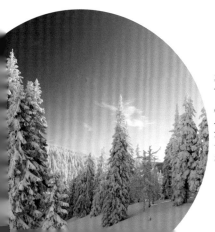

Safety
Use with
caution during
pregnancy.
Possible skin
sensitivity.

1. **Asthma**
*Apply 1-2 drops with carrier oil over chest
or to lung reflex points.*

2. **Immune Stimulant**
Apply 1-2 drops to bottoms of feet.

3. **Dry Cough, Cold, & Flu**
*Inhale 1-2 drops from cupped hands, or
apply with carrier oil over chest.*

4. **Muscle Cramps & Spasms**
*Massage several drops with carrier oil into
affected areas.*

5. **Emotional Overwhelm**
Inhale 1-2 drops from cupped hands.

6. **Rheumatism**
Apply 1-2 drops neat to affected areas.

7. **Mucus**
Apply 1-2 drops to throat and chest.

Single Oils

Spearmint
Mentha Spicata

Application

 A T I

Chemical Constituents
l-carvone
l-limonene
Carveol

Other Uses
Acne, Bronchitis, Headaches, Focus, Migraines, Nervous Fatigue, Respiratory Infection, Sores, Scars

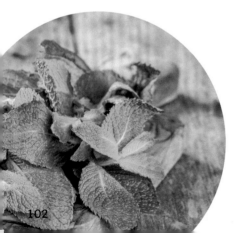

Top *Uses*

1 Indigestion
Drink 1-2 drops in water or in a capsule.

2 Colic
Apply a drop heavily diluted to baby's stomach.

3 Nausea
Inhale 1-2 drops from cupped hands, or rub over stomach.

4 Muscle Aches
Massage 1-2 drops diluted over achy muscles.

5 Bad Breath
Swish 1-2 drops in water as a mouthwash.

6 Heavy Menstruation
Apply 1-2 drops over back of neck and abdomen, or diffuse.

Spikenard
Nardostachys Jatamansi

Application

Chemical Constituents
Jatamansone
Nardol
a-Selinene

Other Uses
Constipation, Depression, Estrogen Imbalance, Fungal Issues, Mental Fatigue, Pinkeye, PMS Cramping, Progesterone Imbalance, Uterus & Ovaries Detox

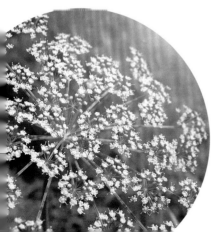

Safety
Use with caution during pregnancy.

Chronic Fatigue Syndrome
Apply 1-2 drops to adrenals and pulse points, or take in a capsule.

Insomnia
Put a drop under the tongue, or take in a capsule.

Toenail Fungus
Apply neat to affected toenail often.

Digestive Inflammation
Take 1-2 drops in a capsule.

Pancreatitis
Apply 1-2 drops neat over pancreas.

Immune Stimulant
Apply 1-2 drops to bottoms of feet.

Hair Loss
Add 2 drops to shampoo, and take 1-2 drops in a capsule.

Single Oils

Tangerine
Citrus Reticulata

Application

Chemical Constituents
d-limonene
B-carotene
Linalol

Other Uses
Anxious Feelings, Chronic Fatigue, Circulation, Detox, Digestive Problems, Muscle Aches, Muscle Spasms, Parasites, Water Retention

Single Oils

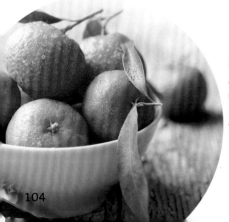

Safety
Avoid sun exposure for 12 hours after topical use.

Top Uses

1 Stress-Induced Insomnia
Inhale 1-2 drops during stressful times of the day. Use a drop under the tongue before bedtime.

2 Cellulite
Massage several drops with carrier oil into cellulite areas.

3 Nervous Exhaustion
Diffuse 4-8 drops, or wear a drop on pulse points.

4 Congestion
Rub 2-4 drops over chest and mid-back.

5 Discouragement
Inhale 1-2 drops from cupped hands. Also add 1-3 drops to water.

6 Flatulence & Constipation
Rub 1-2 drops clockwise over stomach, or drink with water.

Thyme
Thymus Vulgaris

Application
 A T I

Chemical Constituents
Thymol
p-cymene
Linalol

Other Uses
Antioxidant, Asthma, Bites/Stings, Blood Clots, Croup, Eczema/Dermatitis, Fragile Hair, Fungal Infections, Greasy Hair, Hair Loss, Laryngitis, Mold, Numbness, Parasites, Prostatitis, Tendinitis, Tuberculosis

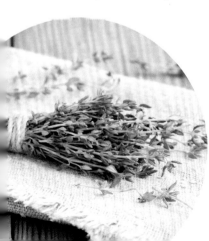

Safety
Possible skin sensitivity. Use with caution during pregnancy or with high blood pressure.

Top Uses

1 Bacterial Infection
Take 1-2 drops in a capsule, or apply to bottoms of feet.

2 Mononucleosis
Take 2 drops in a capsule 3 times daily. Also apply to bottoms of feet.

3 Cough, Cold, & Flu
Diffuse 1-2 drops, and take in a capsule.

4 Bronchitis
Apply 1-2 drops heavily diluted over chest and lung reflex points.

5 Skin Infections
Apply a drop heavily diluted to affected area.

6 Chronic Fatigue
Take 1-2 drops in a capsule, or apply heavily diluted over adrenal glands. Also use one drop in a hot bath.

Turmeric
Curcuma Longa

Application

Chemical Constituents
a-Phellandrene
Terpinolene
1,8-Cineole
p-Cymene
2-Octanol

Other Uses
Arthritis, Blood Sugar, Memory Loss, Weight Loss, Wound Healing

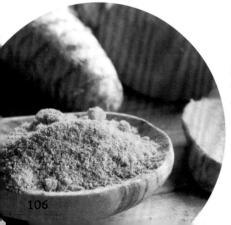

Safety
Contraindicated in pregnancy and infants.

Top *Uses*

1 Chronic Pain & Inflammation
Take 2-4 drops under the tongue or in a veggie capsule. Or rub directly onto location.

2 Heart Palpitations
Rub 2-4 drops over chest; ingest 1-3 drops in a capsule.

3 Tumors
Take 5 drops in a capsule for assistance with tumorous conditions.

4 Brain Function
Take 5 drops in a capsule; rub a drop on the bottoms of big toes.

5 Detoxification
Apply 2 drops to lower back and rib cage.

6 Anxiety & Depression
Diffuse 5 drops to improve mood and obsessive thoughts.

Vetiver
Vetiveria Zizanioides

Application

 A T I

Chemical Constituents
Isovalencenol
a- & B-vetivones
Vitivene

Other Uses
Breast Enlargement, Depression, Irritability, Learning Difficulties, Memory Retention, Muscular Pain, Nerve Issues, Nervous Tension, PMS, Postpartum Depression, Restlessness, Termites, Workaholism

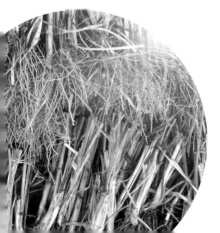

Top *Uses*

1 ADD/ADHD
Apply 1-2 drops behind ears and on the back of the neck.

2 Sleep & Insomnia
Apply 1-2 drops along spine.

3 Skin Irritation
Apply 1-2 drops with carrier oil to affected area.

4 Neuropathy
Apply 1-2 drops to bottoms of feet, or along spine.

5 Balance Issues
Apply 1-2 drops behind ears.

6 Stress-Related Menstrual Issues
Apply 1-2 drops to lower abdomen.

7 PTSD & Anxiety
Apply 1-2 drops behind ears, or diffuse.

Single Oils

Wild Orange
Citrus Sinensis

Application
 ^A ^T ^I

Chemical Constituents
d-Limonene
B-carotene
Citral

Other Uses
Cellulite, Colds, Creativity, Depression, Detox, Fear, Fluid Retention, Heart Palpitations, Insomnia, Menopause, Nervousness, Scurvy, Sluggish Digestion, Withdrawal Issues

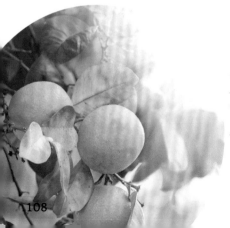

Safety
Avoid sun exposure for 12 hours after topical use.

Top *Uses*

1 Energy
Drink 1-3 drops in water, or inhale from cupped hands.

2 Cheering & Mood Enhancer
Inhale 1-2 drops from cupped hands, or diffuse.

3 Anxiety & Depression
Inhale 1-2 drops from cupped hands, or diffuse 5-10 drops.

4 Immune Support
Gargle 2 drops with water, or apply to bottoms of feet.

5 Sleep Issues
Put a drop under the tongue before bed.

6 Smoothies, Dressings, & Sauces
Add according to taste.

Wintergreen
Gaultheria Procumbens

Application

Chemical Constituents
Methyl Salicylate
Salicylic Acid

Other Uses
Bone Spurs, Cartilage Injury, Circulation,
Muscle Development, Rheumatism

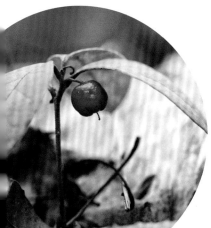

Safety
Potential skin
sensitivity.

1 Muscle Pain & Inflammation
Massage 1-2 drops with carrier oil into affected areas.

2 Arthritis & Gout
Massage 1-2 drops into inflamed joints, diluting if needed.

3 Broken Bones
Apply 1-2 drops gently over injury, avoiding open wounds.

4 Frozen Shoulder & Rotator Cuff
Massage 1-2 drops with carrier oil into affected area.

5 Teeth Whitening
Brush with a drop of oil and baking soda.

6 Dandruff
Add a drop to shampoo, or massage 1-2 drops directly into scalp before shampooing.

Single Oils

Yarrow
Achillea Millefolium

Application

Chemical Constituents
Azulene
Caryophyllene
Pinene

Other Uses
Congestion, Detox, Excess Sodium, Digestive Discomfort, Flatulence, Gallbladder Pain, Headache, Heart Attack, Inflammation, Metabolism, Muscle Spasms, PMS, Weight Loss

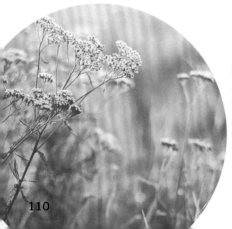

Safety
Can irritate sensitive skin. Avoid long-term use in high doses.

Top Uses

1. Rheumatism & Arthritis
Massage 1-2 drops with carrier oil into affected area.

2. Muscle Injury & Cramps
Massage 1-2 drops into affected area, diluting if needed.

3. Scars
Massage 1-2 drops into scar tissue.

4. Acne
Add a drop to toner or facial cleanser.

5. Varicose Veins
Apply 1-2 drops neat to affected areas.

6. Hemorrhoids
Apply 1-2 drops heavily diluted to affected area.

7. Eczema & Skin Irritation
Apply 1-2 drops diluted to affected area.

Ylang Ylang
Cananga Odorata

Application

Chemical Constituents
B-caryophylle
Benzyl Acetate & Benzoate
Linalol

Other Uses
Anxiety, Arterial Hypertension, Balance Issues, Chronic Fatigue, Circulation, Depression, Diabetes, Exhaustion, Hair Loss, Hypertension, Insomnia, Intestinal Spasms, Tachycardia

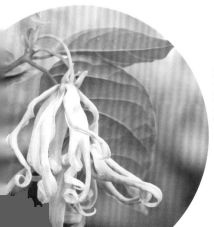

Safety
Dilute for highly sensitive skin.

Hormone Balance
Apply 1-2 drops to wrists and behind ears.

Low Libido
Apply 1-2 drops to pulse points and reproductive reflex points. Diffuse 4-8 drops during intimacy, or use in massage.

High Blood Pressure
Apply 2 drops to bottoms of feet, and take in capsule daily.

Infertility
Massage 1-2 drops over abdomen and reproductive reflex points.

Heart Palpitations
Apply 1-2 drops over heart, and diffuse.

Oily Skin
Add a drop to toner or facial moisturizer, or take 1-2 drops in a capsule daily.

Section 5

Oil
Blends

Anti-Aging Blend

place sticker here

Application

 A T I

Main Ingredients

Frankincense, Sandalwood, Lavender, Myrrh, Helichrysum, Rose

Other Uses

Aging, Blisters, Chapped Skin, Cuts, Dry Skin, Eczema, Hyper-pigmentation, Psoriasis, Sun Burns

Top *Uses*

1. Wrinkles & Fine Lines
   Apply to desired areas morning and night.

2. Age Spots
   Apply to affected areas 3 times daily.

3. Scarring
   Massage for 30 seconds into scar tissue 2-3 times a day until desired appearance.

4. Skin Cancer
   Apply neat to affected area 3x/day.

5. Skin Discoloration
   Apply to affected areas 3 times daily.

6. Meditation
   Apply to pulse points during meditation.

7. Bleeding
   Apply neat to stop minor bleeding.

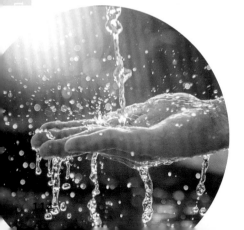

Cellular Complex

Application

 A T I

Main Ingredients
Frankincense, Wild Orange, Lemongrass, Thyme, Summer Savory, Clove, Niaouli

Other Uses
Addictions, Blood Clots, Candida, Cataracts, Fever, Herpes Simplex, Hodgkin's Disease, Glaucoma, Gingivitis, Lipoma, Lupus, Lyme

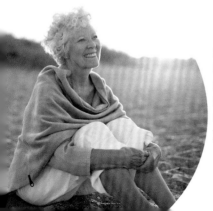

Safety
Can irritate sensitive skin. Use with caution during pregnancy.

Top Uses

1 Thyroid (hypo, Hashimoto's)
Apply diluted over thyroid or to thyroid reflex point, or take 1-2 drops in capsule.

2 Toothache
Apply directly to problematic tooth.

3 Smoking Addiction
Rub onto bottom of big toe.

4 Immune Support
Take 1-2 drops in a capsule.

5 Antioxidant
Take 1-2 drops in a capsule, or use in cooking.

6 Liver Detox
Rub over liver, or on liver reflex point.

7 Rheumatoid Arthritis
Massage diluted into affected area.

Oil Blends

Centering Blend

place sticker / shown name

Application

Main Ingredients

Bergamot, Coriander, Marjoram, Peppermint, Geranium, Basil, Rose, Jasmine

Other Uses

Body Odors, Dizziness, Mood Disorders, Muscle Injury, Nausea, Neuralgia, Vertigo

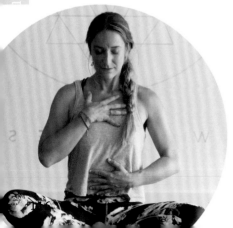

Safety
May cause photosensitivity. Use with caution during pregnancy.

Top Uses

1 Warrior II, Triangle, & Gate Yoga Pose
Apply 2 drops over heart, turning your attention within. Reach inside for power, identity, and assurance.

2 Completeness, Calmness, Courage
Apply 1-3 drops over heart, pulse points, and naval area.

3 Hyperactivity
Apply a drop to temples; diffuse several drops.

4 Addictions
Apply 2-4 drops to bottoms of feet, focusing on big toes; diffuse several drops.

5 Hormone Balancing
Apply 2-4 drops to wrists and inner thighs 2x daily.

6 Neuropathy
Apply 2-4 drops to bottoms of feet 3x daily.

Cleansing Blend

Application

 A T

Main Ingredients
Lime, Lemon, Siberian Fir, Citronella, Melaleuca, Cilantro

Other Uses
Airborne Bacteria & Viruses, Boils, Household Cleaning, Insect Repellent, Mice Repellent, Skin Ulcers

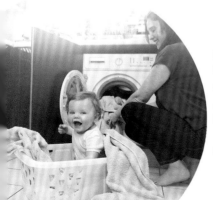

Safety
Can irritate sensitive skin. Avoid direct sun exposure 12 hours after application.

1 Air Freshener
Add 10 drops to glass spray bottle with water. Spray as needed.

2 Foot Odors
Apply neat to feet. Spray inside shoes.

3 Laundry
Add 4-5 drops to detergent.

4 Disinfectant
Add 20 drops to glass spray bottle with water and 1 Tbs rubbing alcohol.

5 Deodorant
Apply 1-2 drops with carrier oil to armpits.

6 Mildew
Use several drops with a clean sponge.

7 Bites & Stings
Apply 1 drop neat to bite or sting.

Oil Blends

117

Comforting Blend

Application

 A   T

Main Ingredients
Frankincense, Ylang Ylang, Patchouli, Labdanum, Sandalwood, Rose, Osmanthus

Other Uses
Anger, Brain Health, Bladder Infection, Emotional Processing, Heart Health, Resentment

Blends

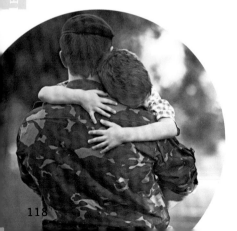

Top Uses

1 Grief, Sorrow, Despair
Apply 1-2 drops over heart, or diffuse.

2 Hormone Balance
Apply 1-2 drops to pulse points before bed.

3 Self-Esteem
Inhale from cupped hands, or diffuse during meditation.

4 Perfume
Wear on pulse points for a floral aroma.

5 Anti-Aging
Apply 1-2 drops with carrier oil to wrinkles, sun spots, and fine lines.

6 Nightmares
Diffuse 3-6 drops next to bedside.

7 Rheumatoid Arthritis
Massage diluted into affected area.

Detoxification Blend

Application

 A   T   I

Main Ingredients
Tangerine, Geranium, Rosemary, Juniper Berry, Cilantro

Other Uses
Hangover, Hormone Balance, Gallbladder Detox, Urinary Infection, Weight Loss

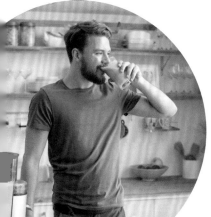

Safety
Can irritate sensitive skin. Avoid sun exposure for 12 hours after topical use.

Top *Uses*

1 Detoxification
Take 1-2 drops in a capsule, or apply to bottoms of feet.

2 Allergies
Apply 1-2 drops to bottoms of feet, or diffuse.

3 Smoking Cravings
Rub onto bottom of big toe, or drink 1-3 drops in water after meals.

4 Liver & Kidney Support
Massage 1-2 drops over liver or kidneys.

5 Antioxidant
Take 1-2 drops in a capsule.

6 Heavy Metal Detox
Apply 1-2 drops to bottoms of feet.

7 Adrenal Fatigue
Massage 1-2 drops over lower back.

Oil Blends

119

Digestive Blend

place sticker *shown name*

Application

 A   T   I

Main Ingredients
Peppermint, Ginger, Caraway, Coriander, Anise, Tarragon

Other Uses
Abdominal Cramps, Acid Reflux, Colitis, Crohn's Disease, Gastritis, Heartburn, Morning Sickness, Motion Sickness, Parasites, Sinusitis

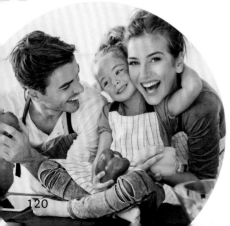

Safety
Can irritate sensitive skin. Use with caution during pregnancy.

Top *Uses*

1 Stomach Upset
Drink 1-2 drops in water, or take in a capsule.

2 Gas & Bloating
Massage 1-2 drops over stomach, or take in a capsule.

3 Diarrhea & Constipation
Massage 1-2 drops over stomach, or take in a capsule.

4 Irritable Bowel Syndrome
Massage 1-2 drops over stomach, or take in a capsule.

5 Food Poisoning
Drink 1-2 drops in water, or take in a capsule.

6 Nausea
Put a drop under the tongue, or rub over stomach.

Encouraging Blend

Application

Main Ingredients
Clementine, Peppermint, Coriander, Basil, Melissa, Rosemary

Other Uses
Asthma, Confusion, Creativity, Fatigue, Loneliness, Overwhelm, Uncertainty

Safety
Can irritate sensitive skin. Use with caution during pregnancy.

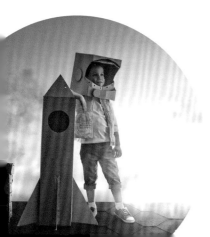

Top *Uses*

1 Discouragement, Low Confidence, Low Motivation
Inhale 1-2 drops from cupped hands, or diffuse.

2 Detox
Apply 1-2 drops to bottoms of feet, or massage over endocrine organs.

3 Adrenal Fatigue
Massage 1-2 drops with carrier oil over lower back.

4 Flatulence
Rub 1-2 drops with carrier oil over stomach.

5 Depression
Diffuse 5-10 drops, or rub 1-2 drops onto temples.

6 Respiratory Issues
Apply 1-2 drops over chest, or diffuse.

Oil Blends

121

Enlightening Blend

Application

 A T I

Main Ingredients
Lemon, Grapefruit, Siberian Fir, Osmanthus, Melissa

Other Uses
Depression, Fear, Respiratory Infection, Sinus Infection, Toxicity, Viral Infection

Blends

Safety
Avoid sun exposure for 12 hours after topical application.

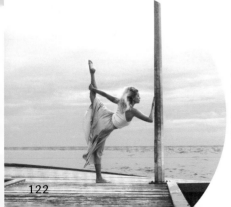

1 Standing Arms High, Standing Side Stretch, & Half Moon Yoga Pose
Apply 2-4 drops to inside of arms and wrists. Feel light entering the crown of your head as your own energy rises to meet it.

2 Lacking Motivation
Apply 1-3 drops to temples and back of neck.

3 Mental Clarity & Illumination
Apply 1-3 drops to temples and forehead.

4 Cold & Flu
Massage 2-4 drops into bottoms of feet and spine; diffuse several drops.

5 Overeating
Massage 2-4 drops over stomach; diffuse several drops.

6 Cold Sores
Apply a drop to affected area 5x daily.

Focus Blend

Application

Main Ingredients
Amyris, Patchouli, Frankincense, Lime, Ylang Ylang, Sandalwood, Chamomile

Other Uses
Alzheimer's, Emotional Balance, Hormone Balance, Memory, Parkinson's, Relaxation, Sleep

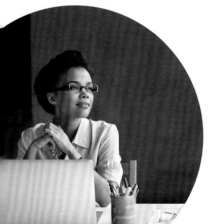

Safety
Repeated use can irritate highly sensitive skin.

1 ADD & ADHD
Apply to back of neck and behind ears.

2 Focus & Concentration
Apply to back of neck and behind ears.

3 Anxiety
Apply to pulse points, or inhale from cupped hands.

4 Hyperactivity
Apply to pulse points, or inhale from cupped hands.

5 Seizures
Apply to bottoms of feet and back of neck.

6 Skin Irritations
Apply with carrier oil to affected areas.

7 Sedative
Apply to pulse points or bottoms of feet.

Oil Blends

Grounding Blend

place sticker
known name

Application

 A   T   I

Main Ingredients
Spruce, Ho Wood, Frankincense, Blue Tansy, Blue Chamomile

Other Uses
Anger, Back Pain, Brain Integration, Bursitis, Comas, Confusion, Convulsions, Diabetic Sores, Grief, Herniated Discs, Hyperactivity, Lou Gehrig's Disease, Parkinson's Disease, Tranquility

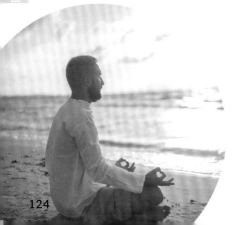

Top Uses

1 Emotional Grounding
Inhale 1-2 drops from cupped hands, or apply to bottoms of feet daily.

2 Focus & Concentration
Apply 1-2 drops to temples and pulse points, or diffuse.

3 Stress & Anxiety
Apply 1-2 drops to pulse points and temples, or to bottoms of feet.

4 Meditation
Apply 1-2 drops to wrists and temples.

5 Neurological Issues
Apply 1-2 drops to bottoms of feet.

6 Stress-Induced Inflammation
Inhale 1-2 drops from cupped hands, apply to bottoms of feet, or diffuse.

7 Balance
Apply 1-2 drops behind ears.

Hopeful Blend

Application

Main Ingredients
Bergamot*, Ylang Ylang, Frankincense, Vanilla

Other Uses
Addictions, Alzheimer's, Appetite Loss, Autism, Discouragement, Parkinson's, Self-Worth Issues

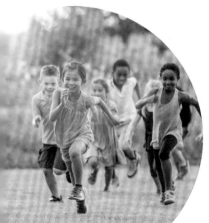

Safety
*FCF Bergamot does not cause photo sensitivity.

1 Emotional Trauma
Apply to pulse points, and inhale from cupped hands.

2 Grief & Trust Issues
Apply to pulse points, and inhale from cupped hands.

3 Hormone Balance
Apply to wrists and bottoms of feet.

4 Perfume
Apply 1-2 drops to pulse points.

5 Adrenal Fatigue
Apply to neck and lower back.

6 Stress
Apply to temples, and inhale from cupped hands.

7 Focus & Concentration
Apply to temples.

Oil Blends

Inspiring Blend

Application

 A   T   I

Main Ingredients
Cardamom, Cinnamon, Ginger, Sandalwood, Jasmine

Other Uses
Depression, Hormone Balance, Menopause, PMS Discomfort, Slow Bowel Movements

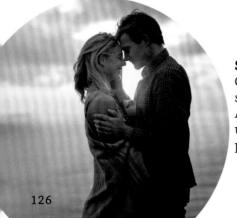

Safety
Can irritate sensitive skin. Avoid topical use during pregnancy.

Top Uses

1 Apathy & Boredom
Inhale 1-2 drops from cupped hands, or diffuse.

2 Low Sex Drive
Apply 1-2 drops with carrier oil to pulse points, or use diluted in massage.

3 Digestive Issues
Apply 1-2 drops to stomach reflex points, or apply diluted over stomach.

4 Aphrodisiac
Apply 1-2 drops to pulse points.

5 Slow Digestion
Apply 1-2 drops with carrier oil over stomach.

6 Lack of Creativity
Diffuse 5-10 drops.

Invigorating Blend

Application

Main Ingredients
Orange, Lemon, Grapefruit, Mandarin, Bergamot, Clementine, Vanilla

Other Uses
Air Freshener, Household Cleaning, Eating Disorders, Laundry Freshener, Low Appetite, Mastitis

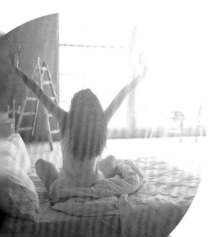

Safety
Avoid sun exposure for 12 hours after topical use.

Top Uses

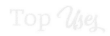

1 Lack of Creativity & Inspiration
Inhale 2 drops from cupped hands, or diffuse.

2 Low Energy
Apply 2 drops to pulse points, or diffuse.

3 Morning Moodiness
Diffuse 5-10 drops next to bedside in the morning, or inhale from cupped hands.

4 Lymphatic Drainage
Apply 3-4 drops to bottoms of feet.

5 Stress & Anxiety
Inhale 2 drops from cupped hands, or apply to pulse points.

6 Depression & Moodiness
Inhale 2 drops from cupped hands, or diffuse 5-10 drops.

Oil Blends

Joyful Blend

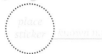

Application

 A T I

Main Ingredients
Lavandin, Lavender, Sandalwood, Tangerine, Melissa, Ylang Ylang, Osmanthus, Lemon Myrtle

Other Uses
Cushing's Syndrome, Lethargy, Postpartum Depression, Sadness, Shock, Weight Loss

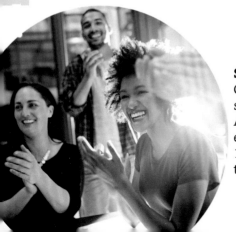

Safety
Can irritate sensitive skin. Avoid sun exposure for 12 hours after topical use.

Blends

Top Uses

1. Depression
Carry on your person, and inhale 1-2 drops from cupped hands as needed.

2. Stress & Anxiety
Diffuse 4-8 drops, or inhale 1-2 drops from cupped hands.

3. Abuse Recovery
Apply 1-2 drops to back of neck and over heart.

4. Grief & Sorrow
Apply 1-2 drops to pulse points, or diffuse.

5. Poison Oak/Ivy
Apply 1-2 drops with carrier oil to affected areas.

6. Lupus & Fibromyalgia
Inhale 1-2 drops from cupped hands, and apply diluted to inflamed areas.

Kids: Courage Blend

Application

 A T I

Main Ingredients
Wild Orange, Amyris, Osmanthus, Cinnamon

Other Uses
Anxiety, Fear, Immune Support, Motivation, Nervousness, Reassurance, Self-Doubt

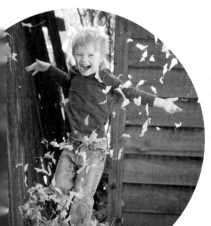

Safety
Avoid sun exposure for 12 hours after topical use.

1 Making New Friends
Apply to wrists and inhale from cupped hands. Speak out loud a few reasons you make a great friend for others!

2 Team Sports
Apply over chest to bring the courage to do your best and be a team player.

3 Potty Training
Apply over lower back and back of neck to feel excited about being a big kid.

4 Electronics Addiction
Apply to wrists and temples to find ambition to experience new adventures.

5 Imagination Sparks
Apply to the back of neck and temples to spur creativity and new ideas.

6 Trying New Things
Apply to the naval and chest to feel brave when trying new things.

Oil Blends

129

Kids: Focus Blend

Application

Main Ingredients
Vetiver, Peppermint, Clementine, Rosemary

Other Uses
Autism, Asperger's, Hyperactivity, Mental Handicaps, Nervous Disorders

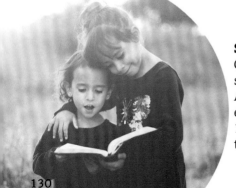

Safety
Can irritate sensitive skin. Avoid sun exposure for 12 hours after topical use.

Top *Uses*

1. Homework
Apply to back of neck at the beginning of homework time to boost concentration.

2. ADD/ADHD
Apply to the back of neck 3x daily or as needed.

3. Creative Writing
Apply to temples to incite new ideas during writing projects.

4. Household Chores
Apply to naval and wrists to stay focused during chore time so that playtime can come sooner.

5. Test Taking
Apply to temples while studying for a test, and again while taking the test.

6. Confusion & Distractions
Apply to temples and inhale from cupped hands to promote mental clarity.

Application

Main Ingredients
Amyris, Balsam Fir, Coriander, Magnolia

Other Uses
Chronic Pain, Circulation Issues, Cough, Cramps, Depression, Procrastination, Scrapes, Stress

1 Social Anxiety
Apply to wrists and lower back to add a feeling of steadiness to social situations.

2 Frazzled School Mornings
Start the morning right by applying to bottoms of feet and the back of the neck.

3 Useful Time-Outs
Turn time-outs from unhelpful punishment to a time of valuable reflection on the importance of keeping your word and contributing value to the family.

4 Superhero Confidence
Apply over chest and the back of neck.

5 Waaaah-Baby
Apply to temples and wrists to calm temper tantrums.

6 Bad News Buster
Apply over chest to help ease disappointment or discouragement.

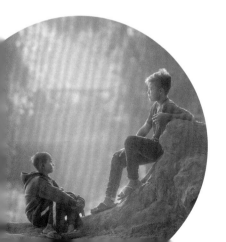

Oil Blends

131

Kids: Protective Blend

place sticker / generic name

Application

 A   T   I

Main Ingredients
Cedarwood, Litsea, Frankincense, Rose

Other Uses
Athlete's Foot, Dandruff, Fungal Infection, Heartache, Ingrown Toenail

Blends

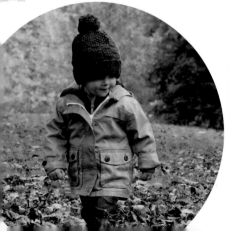

Safety
Can irritate highly sensitive skin.

Top *Uses*

1 Playtime-Ready
Rub on hands, back of neck, and under nose to ward off germs during play with other kids.

2 Cold & Flu
Apply to chest, spine, and bottoms of feet 5x daily.

3 Super Hero Immunity
Apply to bottoms of feet each morning for immune system boost.

4 Zombie Attacks (Bacteria, Virus, Fungus)
Apply 3-5x daily to infected areas.

5 Fatigue
Apply over kidneys and adrenals 2x daily to improve stamina.

6 Inner Circle Friends
Inhale from cupped hands to remember maintaining healthy boundaries and respect in friendships.

Kids: Restful Blend

Application

 A T

Main Ingredients
Lavender, Cananga, Buddha Wood, Roman Chamomile

Other Uses
Behavioral Disorders, Bee Sting, Crying, Diaper Rash, Hyperactivity, Hyper-pigmentation, Neuralgia, Shock, Spider Bite, Sunburn, Worms

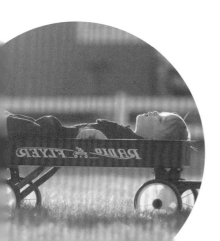

1 Easy Sleeping
Apply to bottoms of feet and back of neck 30 minutes before bedtime for an easier time falling asleep.

2 Monsters in the Closet
Apply over chest and wrists to ease nighttime fears.

3 Argument Diffuser
Apply to temples and back of neck to ease contention.

4 Tornado Thoughts
Apply to temples, wrists, and back of neck to soothe runaway and irrational thoughts.

5 Grown-Up Relaxation
Apply liberally to temples and chest before getting into a warm bath to let go of a stressful day of kid's duties.

Oil Blends

Kids: Soothing Blend

Application

 A T I

Main Ingredients
Copaiba, Lavender, Spearmint, Zanthoxylum

Other Uses
Charley Horse, Growing Pains, Headache, Lethargy, Joint Pain, Muscle Pain, Muscle Tension

Safety
Can irritate sensitive skin. Use with caution during pregnancy.

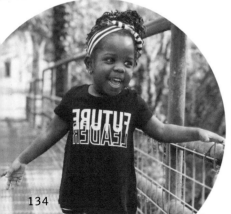

Top *Uses*

1 Battle Wounds
Apply liberally to ease pain and injury that happen with the dangers of being an active kid.

2 Sports Injury
Apply to injured muscles, joints, and connective tissue 5x daily.

3 Bumps & Bruises
Apply every couple hours to reduce the appearance of bruises or bumps.

4 Self-Trust
Apply to the back of neck and temples to remember the power of trusting your good instincts.

5 Stinky Feet
Apply to feet before and after school.

6 Mighty Muscles
Apply to legs, arms, and shoulders as a pre-workout before sports and exercise.

Blends

Massage Blend

Application

Main Ingredients

Cypress, Peppermint, Marjoram, Basil, Grapefruit, Lavender

Other Uses

Arthritis, Circulation, Ligament Damage, Muscular Dystrophy, Relaxation, Tension

Safety
Can irritate sensitive skin. Use with caution during pregnancy.

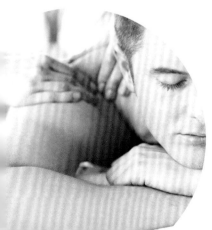

Top Uses

1. Muscle Tension & Aches
Massage 2-4 drops with carrier oil into tight muscles.

2. Adrenal Fatigue & Lethargy
Apply 1-2 drops to lower back.

3. Back, Neck, & Shoulder Pain
Massage 2-4 drops with carrier oil into affected muscles, or add to hot bath.

4. Post-Work Stress
Massage 2 drops into back of neck to relieve stress from work.

5. Neuropathy
Apply 1-2 drops to bottoms of feet.

6. High Blood Pressure
Apply 1-2 drops to bottoms of feet.

7. Headache
Apply 1-2 drops to temples, avoiding eyes.

Metabolic Blend

place sticker of known vials

Application
 A T I

Main Ingredients
Grapefruit, Lemon, Ginger, Peppermint, Cinnamon

Other Uses
Colds, Congestion, Detox, Energy, Food Addiction, Gallbladder Stones, High Cholesterol, Lymphatic Stimulation, Obesity, Over-Eating

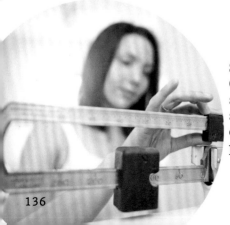

Safety
Can irritate sensitive skin. Use with caution during pregnancy.

Top *Uses*

1 Weight Loss
Take 2-4 drops in capsule or drink in water.

2 Appetite Control
Drink 2-4 drops in water throughout the day, or diffuse.

3 Blood Sugar Regulation
Take 1-2 drops in water or in a capsule.

4 Cellulite & Visceral Fat
Massage several drops with carrier oil into needed areas.

5 Antioxidant
Take 1-2 drops in a capsule.

6 Eating Disorders
Take a drop under the tongue, or diffuse 4-8 drops.

Outdoor Blend

Application

Main Ingredients

Catnip, Skimmia Laureola, Amyris, Balsam, Orange, White Fir, Eucalyptus, African Sandalwood, Genet, Rose

Other Uses

Ants, Mites, Termites, Tics

1 **Insect Repellent**
Apply directly to exposed skin, and diffuse if possible

2 **Fly Infestation**
Diffuse 10 drops, or apply lightly over clothing.

3 **Energetic Toxicity**
Use 1-3 drops during meditation, journaling, or prayer.

Oil Blends

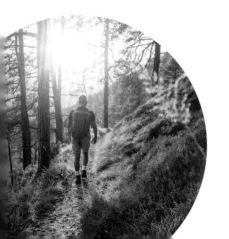

Protective Blend

Application

 A T I

Main Ingredients

Orange, Clove, Cinnamon, Rosemary, Eucalyptus

Other Uses

Autoimmune Disorders, Cough, Germs, Household Cleaning, Hypoglycemia, Laundry Booster, Mold, Pneumonia, Staph Infection, Strep Throat, Warts

Safety
Can irritate sensitive skin. Use with caution during pregnancy.

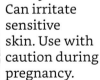

Top *Uses*

1 Immune Support
Take 1-2 drops in capsule as daily supplement, or apply to bottoms of feet.

2 Colds & Flu
Apply 1-2 drops to bottoms of feet, and take with water or in a capsule.

3 Airborne Viruses
Diffuse 5-10 drops.

4 Mouthwash
Rinse mouth with 2 drops and water.

5 Cold Sores
Apply a drop with carrier oil to needed areas.

6 MRSA
Apply 1-2 drops diluted to affected areas.

7 Gum Disease & Cavities
Rinse mouth with 2 drops and water.

Reassuring Blend

Application

 A T I

Main Ingredients
Vetiver, Lavender, Ylang Ylang, Frankincense, Marjoram, Spearmint, Labdanum

Other Uses
Addictive Personality, Postpartum Recovery, Social Anxiety

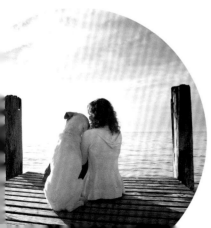

Safety
Use with caution during beginning of pregnancy.

1 Fear & Insecurity
Apply 1-2 drops over temples or chest.

2 Worry
Inhale 1-2 drops from cupped hands.

3 Restlessness & Irritability
Apply 1-2 drops to temples or bottoms of feet, or diffuse.

4 Sleep Issues
Diffuse 4-8 drops near bedside, or apply 1-2 drops to temples.

5 Focus Issues
Apply 1-2 drops to back of neck or temples.

6 Social Disorders
Inhale 1-2 drops from cupped hands, or rub onto back of neck.

Oil Blends

Renewing Blend

Application

Main Ingredients
Spruce, Bergamot, Juniper Berry, Myrrh, Arborvitae, Citronella, Thyme, Nootka

Other Uses
Bitterness, Emotional Stagnation, Kidney Stones, Liver Issues, Muscle Pain, Sadness, Shame, Skin Infection

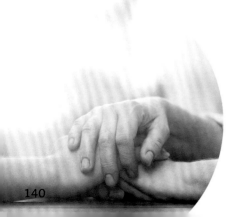

Top Uses

1 **Anger, Resentment, Guilt**
Apply 1-2 drops to pulse points, and inhale from cupped hands.

2 **Attachment Issues**
Apply 1-2 drops to pulse points, and diffuse.

3 **Critical Thinking**
Apply 1-2 drops to temples and back of neck, and diffuse.

4 **Circulation**
Apply 2-4 drops to bottoms of feet.

5 **Insect Repellent**
Apply with carrier oil over exposed skin.

6 **Prostate Issues**
Apply 1-2 drops over lower abdomen.

7 **Irritability**
Inhale 1-2 drops from cupped hands.

Blends

Respiratory Blend

Application

 A T I

Main Ingredients
Laurel, Eucalyptus, Peppermint, Melaleuca, Lemon, Cardamom, Ravintsara

Other Uses
Constricted Breathing, Emphysema, Exercise-Induced Asthma, Nasal Polyps, Respiratory Infections, Sinusitis, Tuberculosis

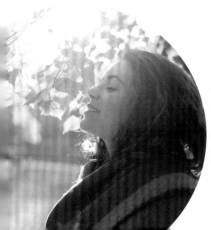

Safety
Can irritate sensitive skin. Use with caution during pregnancy.

1 Cough, Bronchitis, Pneumonia
Inhale 2-4 drops from cupped hands, and apply diluted over chest.

2 Asthma
Inhale 2-4 drops from cupped hands, and apply to lung reflex points.

3 Cold & Flu
Diffuse 5-10 drops, or apply with carrier oil over chest.

4 Allergies
Apply 1-2 drops over bridge of nose and sinuses, avoiding eyes.

5 Snoring
Apply 1-2 drops over throat and bridge of nose, avoiding eyes.

6 Closed off from Love
Rub a few drops over heart.

Oil Blends

Restful Blend

Application

Main Ingredients

Lavender, Sweet Marjoram, Chamomile, Ylang Ylang, Sandalwood, Cedarwood, Vetiver, Vanilla

Other Uses

Addictions, Hyperactivity, Insomnia, Lock Jaw, Mental Fatigue, Temporomandibular Joint Disorder (TMJ), Tension

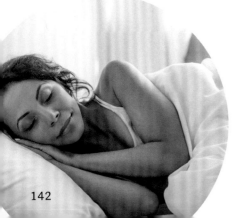

Safety
Use with caution during pregnancy.

Top Uses

1 Sleep Issues
Apply 1-2 drops to temples and bottoms of feet, and diffuse near bedside.

2 Stress & Anxiety
Apply 1-2 drops to pulse points, and inhale from cupped hands.

3 ADD & ADHD
Apply 1-2 drops to back of neck, and diffuse.

4 Itchy Skin
Apply 1-2 drops with carrier oil to affected areas.

5 Anger & Restlessness
Massage 1-2 drops into back of neck.

6 Hormone Balance & Mood Swings
Apply 1-2 drops to pulse points, or diffuse.

Skin Clearing Blend

Application

Main Ingredients

Black Cumin, Ho Wood, Melaleuca, Geranium, Eucalyptus, Litsea

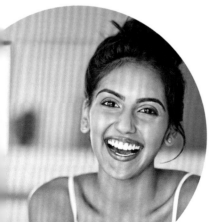

Safety
Possible skin irritation.

Top Uses

1. Acne & Blemishes
   Apply directly to areas of concern.

2. Skin Impurities
   Rub into skin before washing.

3. Oily Skin
   Apply to areas of concern.

4. Eczema & Dermatitis
   Apply with carrier oil to affected areas.

5. Bacterial Infection
   Apply to affected areas.

143

Soothing Blend

place sticker of bottle here

Application

 A   T   I

Main Ingredients

Wintergreen, Camphor, Peppermint, Blue Tansy, Helichrysum, Blue Chamomile

Other Uses

Back Pain, Bursitis, Frozen Shoulder, Growing Pains, Injured Joints, Tendinitis, Tennis Elbow, Workout (Pre and Post)

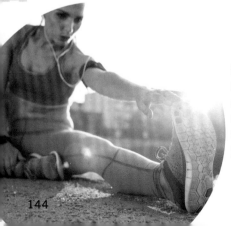

Safety

Can irritate sensitive skin. Use with caution during pregnancy.

Top Uses

1 Muscle Pain & Inflammation
Massage 2-4 drops with carrier oil or lotion into affected areas.

2 Joint Pain & Arthritis
Apply 1-2 drops to affected areas.

3 Lupus & Fibromyalgia
Apply 1-2 drops with carrier oil when experiencing flare-ups.

4 Whiplash
Apply 2-4 drops to affected areas.

5 Bruises
Gently apply 1-2 drops to bruising.

6 Headache
Apply 1-2 drops to temples and back of neck.

7 Bone Pain
Apply 2-4 drops directly over pain.

Steadying Blend

Application

Main Ingredients
Lavender, Cedarwood, Frankincense, Cinnamon, Sandalwood, Black Pepper, Patchouli

Other Uses
Agitation, Bipolar Disorder, Calming, Courage, Muscle Fatigue, Sleep Issues

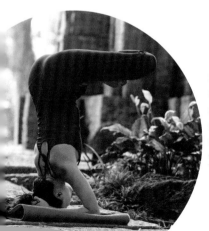

Safety
Can irritate sensitive skin. Use with caution during pregnancy.

Top *Uses*

1 Seated Meditation, Seated Twist, & Bhu Mudra yoga poses
Apply a couple drops to heels, over ears, and the base of skull.

2 Circulation Issues
Apply 2-4 drops to the bottoms of feet morning and evening.

3 Muscle Spasms
Massage 2-4 drops into the bottoms of feet and into affected muscles.

4 Energetic Focus
Apply a drop to temples and inhale from cupped hands to center your attention.

5 Emotional Numbness
Massage 2-4 drops into sacral area and lower spine.

6 Cracked or Chapped Skin
Massage 2-4 drops with extra FCO into affected areas.

Tension Blend

Application

 A T I

Main Ingredients

Wintergreen, Lavender, Peppermint, Frankincense, Cilantro, Marjoram, Chamomile, Rosemary

Other Uses

Alertness, Calming, Inflammation, Muscle Cramps, Swelling

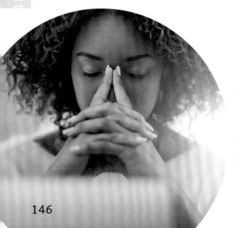

Safety

Can irritate sensitive skin. Use with caution during pregnancy.

1 Headache & Migraine
Massage into temples and forehead, avoiding eyes.

2 Muscle Tension
Massage into areas of concern.

3 Hot Flashes
Apply to back of neck.

4 Fevers
Apply to back of neck.

5 Bruises
Apply gently over bruises.

6 Hangover
Apply to temples and over stomach.

7 Arthritis
Massage into aching joints.

146

Uplifting Blend

Application

Main Ingredients
Orange, Clove, Star Anise, Lemon Myrtle, Nutmeg, Ginger, Cinnamon, Zdravetz

Other Uses
Digestive Discomfort, Food Addiction, Jaw Pain, Lock Jaw, Low Energy

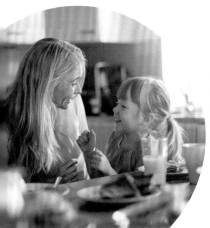

Safety
Can irritate sensitive skin. Use with caution during pregnancy.

1 Gloominess
Inhale 1-2 drops from cupped hands.

2 Self-Sabotage
Apply 1-2 drops over naval, and diffuse.

3 Low Energy
Apply 1-2 drops over adrenals on lower back, and diffuse.

4 Pessimism
Apply 1-2 drops to pulse points, and diffuse.

5 Detoxification
Apply 2-4 drops to bottoms of feet.

6 Emotional Disconnect
Apply 1-2 drops to temples or over heart.

7 Moodiness
Apply 1-2 drops to pulse points, or diffuse.

Oil Blends

147

Women's Monthly Blend

place sticker of blend here

Application

Main Ingredients

Clary Sage, Lavender, Bergamot, Chamomile, Cedarwood, Ylang Ylang, Geranium, Fennel, Carrot Seed, Palmarosa, Vitex

Other Uses

Aphrodisiac, Sedative, Sleep Issues

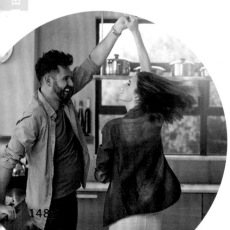

Safety
Avoid sun exposure for 12 hours after topical use.

Top Uses

1 PMS
Apply to wrists and over lower abdomen.

2 Cramping
Apply to lower abdomen.

3 Hormone Balance
Apply to wrists and over lower abdomen.

4 Hot Flashes
Apply to wrists and back of neck.

5 Mood Swings
Inhale from cupped hands, and apply to pulse points.

6 Self-Confidence
Inhale from cupped hands, and apply to pulse points.

7 Heavy Menstruation
Apply to lower abdomen.

Blends

148

Women's Perfume Blend

Application

Main Ingredients

Bergamot, Ylang Ylang, Patchouli, Jasmine, Vanilla, Cinnamon, Labdanum, Vetiver, Cocoa, Rose

Other Uses

Loss of Vision, Skin Irritation

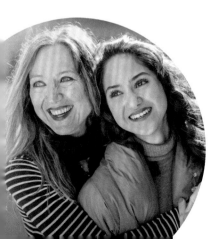

1 Perfume
Apply 1-2 drops to pulse points.

2 Hormone Balance
Apply 1-2 drops to pulse points and back of neck.

3 Aphrodisiac
Apply 1-2 drops to neck and wrists.

4 Sedative & Calming
Inhale 1-2 drops from cupped hands.

5 Low Sex Drive
Apply 1-2 drops to pulse points.

6 Menopause
Apply 1-2 drops to pulse points.

Section 6

Supplements
& Softgels

Vitality Supplement Set (trio)

place sticker *known name*

Components
- Cellular Vitality Complex
- Essential Oil + Omegas
- Food Nutrient Complex

Key Uses
- Vitality & Wellness
- Immune System Support
- Pain & Inflammation
- Sleep
- Mood, Depression, Anxiety
- Energy
- Hormone Balance
- Provides bio-available crucial nutrients to cells for building healthy organs, tissues, and body systems.

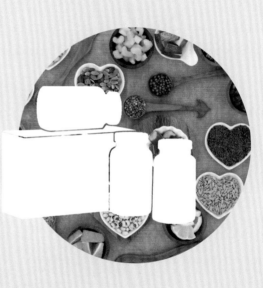

Supplements

Bone Nutrient

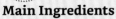

Main Ingredients
Calcium (coral calcium), Vitamin C, Vitamin D-2, Biotin, Magnesium, Zinc, Copper, Manganese, Boron

Key Uses
- Promotes Bone Health
- Prevents age-related calcium loss
- Maintains bone mineralization
- Maximizes calcium utilization

Cellular Complex Softgel

Main Ingredients
Frankincense, Orange, Lemongrass, Thyme, Summer Savory, Niaouli, Clove

Key Uses
- Aids in elimination of unhealthy cells
- Facilitates DNA repair
- Promotes healthy cellular function
- Useful for cancer, tumors, inflammation, infections, nervous system issues, immune system issues

Cellular Vitality Complex

Main Ingredients
Boswellia Serrata, Scuttelaria Root, Milk Thistle, Pineapple Extract, Polygonum Capsudatum, Tumeric Root, Red Rasperry, Grape Seed, Marigold Flower, Tomato Fruit

Key Uses
- Protects body against free radicals
- Maintains proper cellular function
- Improves cellular vitality & energy
- Reduces inflammation

Children's Chewable

Main Ingredients
Vitamins A, C, D, E, B1, B2, B3, B6, B12, B5, Folic Acid, Biotin, Calcium, Iron, Iodine, Magnesium, Zinc, Copper, Manganese, Superfood Blend, Cellular Vitality Blend

Key Uses
- Complete daily nutrient for children
- Food-derived nutrients
- Easy to ingest
- Pairs perfectly with other supplements

Supplements

Children's Omega-3

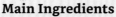
place sticker, known name

Main Ingredients
Fish Oil (EPA, DHA), Vitamin D, Vitamin E, Vitamin C, Orange Essential Oil

Key Uses
- Provides benefits of fish oil without fishy taste
- Easy to take plain, or add to juice
- Supports brain, joint, and cardiovascular development

Children's Probiotic

place sticker, known name

Main Ingredients
Lactobacillus Rhamnosus, Lactobacillus Salivarius, Lactobaccilus Plantarum LP01 & LP02, Bifidobacterium Breve, Bifidobacterium Lactis

Key Uses
- 5 billion live cells of 6 strains of flora
- Supports healthy digestive, neurological, immune, and brain function
- Shelf-stable unique delivery process

Daily Supplement (duo)

place sticker, known name

Components
Food Nutrient Complex, Essential Oil + Omegas

Key Uses
- Provides complete daily nutrients derived from whole foods
- Complex omegas without standard preservatives, combined with essential oils
- Bioavailable nutrients to support body systems, organs, and cellular health

Detox Herbal Complex

place sticker, known name

Main Ingredients
Psyllium Seed Husk, Barberry Leaf, Turkish Rhubarb, Kelp, Milk Thistle, Osha Root, Safflower, Acacia Gum, Burdoc, Root, Clove, Enzyme Assimilation Complex

Key Uses
- Whole-food Detox Herbal Complex
- Promotes healthy endocrine system
- Promotes toxin filtration
- Compliments Detoxification Blend

154

Detoxification Softgels

Main Ingredients
Tangerine, Rosemary, Geranium, Juniper Berry, Cilantro

Key Uses
- Endocrine Support
- Promotes release of toxins
- Hormone Balance
- Antioxidant
- Stimulates adrenals
- Cleanses filtration organs

Digestion Comfort Tablets

Main Ingredients
Calcium Carbonate, Ginger, Fennel, Coriander, Peppermint, Tarragon, Anise, Caraway

Key Uses
- Soothes GI discomfort
- Relieves heartburn and indigestion
- Relieves sour stomach
- Reduces belching and bloating

Digestive Enzymes

Main Ingredients
Protease, Amylase, Lipase, Alpha Galactosidase, Cellulase, Maltase, Sucrase, Tummy Taming Blend, Enzyme Assimilation Blend

Key Uses
- Facilitates breakdown of food
- Increases nutrient absorption
- Promotes comfortable digestion
- Increases usability of nutrients
- Facilitates proper gut function

Digestive Blend Softgels

Main Ingredients
Ginger, Peppermint, Tarragon, Fennel, Caraway, Coriander, Anise

Key Uses
- Soothes digestive discomfort
- Reduces gas and flatulence
- Reduces nausea
- Reduces diarrhea and constipation

Supplements

155

Energy & Stamina Complex

 known name

Main Ingredients
Acetyl-L-Carnitine, Alpha-Lipolic Acid, Co-enzyme Q10, Lychee Fruit, Green Tea Leaf, Quercetine Dihydrate, Cordyceps Mycelium, Ginseng, Ashwagandha

Key Uses
· Increases cellular energy
· Improves micro-circulation
· Stimulates mitochondria
· Improves stamina

Essential Oil + Omegas

 known name

Main Ingredients
Fish Oil (EPA DHA), Astaxanthin, Flaxseed Oil, Borage Seed Oil, Cranberry Seed Oil, Pomegranate Seed Oil, Vitamin D

Key Uses
· Promotes heart, brain, joint, eye, skin, and circulatory health
· Protects against lipid oxidation
· Molecularly filtered fish oil combined with internal dose of 9 essential oils

Food Nutrient Complex

 known name

Main Ingredients
Vitamins A, C, D, E, K, B6, B12, Thiamin, Riboflavin, Niacin, Folate, Biotin, Pantothenic Acid, Calcium, Iron, Iodine, Magnesium, Zinc, Selenium, Copper, Manganese

Key Uses
· Whole-food comprehensive vitamin and mineral nutrient
· Provides bioavailable crucial nutrients to body systems, organs, and cells

Fruit & Veggie Drink Mix

 known name

Main Ingredients
Kale, Dandelion, Collard Greens, Wheat Grass, Alfalfa, Barley Grass, Goji Berry, Mangosteen, Lemon & Ginger Oil

Key Uses
· Provides essential nutrients
· Supports Immune Health
· Supports Digestive Health
· Supports Weight Loss
· All natural ingredients

Supplements

GI Cleansing Complex

Main Ingredients
Caprylic Acid; Oregano, Melaleuca, Lemon, Lemongrass, and Thyme Oils

Key Uses
- Helps rid gut of parasites, Candida, and other harmful agents
- Supports healthy digestive environment
- Helps improve microbial balance

Phytoestrogen Complex

Main Ingredients
Soy Extract (64% isoflavones, 50% Genistein), Flaxseed Extract (40% Lignan), Pomegranate Extract (40% Ellagic Acid)

Key Uses
- Promotes hormone balance by blocking estrogen binding to cells
- Manages harmful metabolite byproducts of hormone metabolism

Polyphenol Complex

Main Ingredients
Frankincense Extract, Turmeric, Ginger, Green Tea Extract, Pomegranate Extract, Grape Seed Extract, Resveratrol

Key Uses
- Reduces inflammation and pain
- Provides relief to tension headaches, as well as back, neck, and shoulder pain
- Antioxidant support
- Internal compliment to Soothing Blend

Probiotic Complex

Main Ingredients
L. acidophilus, B. lactis, L. salivarius, L. casei, B. longum, B. bifidum

Key Uses
- 6 billion CFUs
- Supports digestive & immune systems
- Unique double-encapsulated delivery
- Shelf stable with prebiotics to sustain probiotics
- Helps digestion of food nutrients

Supplements

Protective Softgels +

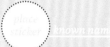
place sticker *known name*

Main Ingredients
Clove, Wild Orange, Black Pepper, Cinnamon, Eucalyptus, Oregano, Rosemary, Melissa

Key Uses
• Supercharged Protective Blend
• Combats viral and bacterial infections
• Supports immune system

Restful Complex

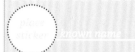
place sticker *known name*

Main Ingredients
Lavender, L-theanine, Lemonbalm, Passion Flower, Chamomile

Key Uses
• Promotes falling asleep faster
• Supports more meaningful sleep
• Promotes waking up feeling refreshed

Seasonal Blend Softgels

place sticker *known name*

Main Ingredients
Lemon, Lavender, & Peppermint Essential Oils

Key Uses
• Reduces histamine response
• Opens airways
• Relieves itchiness
• Eases sinus congestion
• Useful for seasonal and pet allergies

Trim Shake

place sticker *known name*

Main Ingredients
Whey & Egg White Protein, Fiber Blend, Stevia, Annatto, Ashwagandha, Potato Protein, Trim Complex

Key Uses
• Meal replacement shake
• Reduces cortisol levels to reduce fat retention
• Manages appetite and cravings
• Healthy protein-carb-fat ratio

Supplements

Section 7

Protocols

Acne (bacteria)

Description
Combats bacterial over-growth that becomes trapped in pores.

Suggested Duration
Ongoing

Skin Clearing Blend
Apply a small amount evenly over clean skin after showering daily.

Melaleuca & Lavender
Apply a dab to blemishes.

Frankincense
Apply a dab to healing blemishes to prevent scarring.

Additional Support
• Anti-Aging Blend
• Helichrysum

Acne (hormones)

Description
Balances hormone production and maintenance throughout the body, including the gut.

Suggested Duration
Until desired appearance is achieved, then as needed

Vitality Supplement Trio
Take 2 of each supplement twice daily.

Phytoestrogen Complex
Take 1 capsule with each dose of Vitality Supplements (for men and women).

Clary Sage
Rub 1 drop on pulse points before bed.

Skin Clearing Blend
Apply a small amount to blemishes daily as needed.

Acne (toxicity)

Description
Alleviates toxicity overload by detoxing organs and skin.

Suggested Duration
3-5 weeks

Detoxification Softgels
Take 1 softgel with each meal.

Detox Herbal Complex
Take 1 capsule with breakfast and dinner.

Cellular Complex Softgels
Take 1 softgel with each meal.

Skin Clearing Blend
Apply small amount to blemishes daily as needed.

Additional Support
• GI Cleansing Complex
• Helichrysum
• Detoxification Blend (use on bottoms of feet)

ADD/ADHD

Description

Designed to activate the parasympathetic nervous system and induce a more calm and focused mental state.

Suggested Duration

6 months, then as needed

Vetiver, Frankincense, Rose

Apply 1-2 drops of each oil to back of neck, spine and bottoms of feet 2x daily.

Focus Blend

Carry in your pockct, and roll a small amount on back of neck as needed for focus.

Probiotic Complex

Take 2 capsules in the morning on an empty stomach.

Additional Support

• Ylang Ylang
• Sandalwood
• Roman Chamomile

Adrenal Fatigue

Description

Supports healthy adrenal function.

Suggested Duration

4-8 weeks

Lemon (8), **Basil** (3), **Rosemary** (3), **Frankincense** (3)
Combine in roller bottle. Fill the rest with carrier oil. Massage into neck and kidneys daily as often as needed.

Rosemary & Peppermint

Breathe a drop of each from cupped hands, or diffuse for energy as needed.

Vitality Supplement Trio

Take 2 of each bottle 2x daily.

Energy & Stamina Complex

Take 2 capsules 2x daily.

Additional Support

• Invigorating Blend
• Detoxification Blend

AIDS/HIV

Description

Provides emotional support, promotes a properly functioning immune system.

Suggested Duration

6 months, then as needed

Cellular Complex Blend

Rub 3-5 drops onto spine morning & night.

Cellular Complex Softgels

Take 2 softgels 3x daily.

Vitality Supplement Trio

Take 2 of each bottle 2x daily.

Protective Blend & Melissa

Rub 2 drops each on bottoms of feet 2x daily.

Joyful Blend

Carry with you, and inhale from hands for emotional support throughout the day.

Protocols

Allergies (food)

Description
Lowers histamine response triggered by food allergies and creates calm in the gut.

Suggested Duration
4 weeks to begin, then as needed

Lavender
Put 1 drop under tongue. Drink water after 30 seconds.

Probiotic Complex
Take 1 capsule 3x daily on an empty stomach.

Polyphenol Complex
Take 1 capsule 3x daily.

Digestive Enzyme Complex
Take 1 with each meal.

Additional Support
• Do a 14-day bone broth cleanse
• Detox Herbal Complex
• Detoxification Blend

Allergies (pet/seasonal)

Description
Reduces histamine response and boosts immune response.

Suggested Duration
4-8 weeks, then as needed

Lemon, Lavender, Peppermint
Put 1 drop each under tongue. Drink water after 30 seconds.

Respiratory Blend
Inhale from cupped hands when experiencing attack.

Probiotic Complex
Take 1 capsule 3x daily on an empty stomach.

Protective Blend
Gargle 2 drops with water nightly, then swallow.

Additional Support
• Seasonal Blend Softgels
• Siberian Fir
• Vitality Supplement Trio

Allergies (skin)

Description
Calms irritation due to skin contact with allergens.

Suggested Duration
As needed

Lavender, Helichrysum, Frankincense, Lemon
Combine 10 drops of each in a roller bottle. Fill the rest with carrier oil. Roll onto affected area often.

Lavender
Put a drop under tongue. Drink water after 30 seconds.

Probiotic Complex
Take 1 capsule 3x daily on an empty stomach.

Additional Support
• Detox Herbal Complex
• Detoxification Blend

Alzheimer's

Supports healthy mental activity, boosts alertness.

Ongoing

Vitality Supplement Trio
Take 2 of each bottle 2x daily.

Cellular Complex Blend
Rub 3-5 drops along spine and bottoms of feet 3x daily.

Cellular Complex Softgels
Take 1 softgel 3x daily.

Peppermint & Rosemary
Massage a drop each into scalp and diffuse several drops daily to increase alertness & memory.

• Cilantro
• Frankincense
• Extra Omega Complex
• Grounding Blend

Anxiety

Increases a general calming state due to the interaction of oils with neurotransmitters.

3 months, then as needed

Roman Chamomile, Lavender, Vetiver
Apply a drop of each to back of neck, spine, and bottoms of feet 3x daily.

Focus Blend
Apply to temples and sides of neck 3x daily.

Probiotic Complex
Take 2 capsules in the morning on an empty stomach.

Magnolia
Roll over back of neck 3x daily and as needed.

• Frankincense

Arthritis

Decreases the inflammatory response within the joint tissues.

6 months, then as needed

Copaiba, Turmeric, Frankincense
Apply a drop of each to affected areas 3x daily.

Soothing Blend
Massage lotion into affected areas after above oils 3x daily.

Polyphenol Complex
Take 2 capsules in the evening with food.

• Marjoram
• Lemongrass
• Wintergreen
• Myrrh

Asthma

Description
Promotes open airways and easy breathing.

Suggested Duration
As needed

Respiratory Blend
Inhale 2 drops from cupped hands during attacks.

Lavender
Massage a drop behind and over ears to promote calm.

Cardamom
Gargle a drop for 30 seconds, then swallow as needed.

Probiotic Complex
Take 1 capsule 2x daily.

Additional Support
· Rosemary
· Siberian Fir
· Eucalyptus

Autism

Description
Increases the integrity of the gut lining and promotes brain health.

Suggested Duration
1 to 3 years

Frankincense, Vetiver, Turmeric, Clary Sage
Apply a drop of each diluted to back of neck and bottoms of feet 3x daily.

Cellular Complex & Rose
Apply 2 drops each diluted to spine 2x daily.

Probiotic Complex
Take 2 capsules in the morning on an empty stomach.

Lavender, Melaleuca, Frankincense, Digestive Blend, Copaiba
Roll diluted clockwise over stomach 2x daily.

Digestive Enzymes
Take 1 capsule with each meal.

Back, Neck, Shoulder Pain

Description
Increases circulation, reduces scar tissue, promotes healing.

Suggested Duration
6-12 months

Frankincense, Turmeric, Copaiba
Take a drop of each in a capsule or under the tongue 3x daily.

Polyphenol Complex
Take 2 capsules 2x daily on an empty stomach.

Marjoram, Frankincense, Lemongrass, Siberian Fir, Soothing Blend (lotion)
Apply a drop of each onto spine and painful areas 3x daily.

Additional Support
· Yarrow

Bipolar Disorder

Description
Normalizes brain activity and regulates nervous system.

Suggested Duration
12 months

Frankincense, Vetiver, Turmeric, Clary Sage
Apply a drop of each to back of neck and bottoms of feet 2x daily.

Cellular Complex
Apply 2-4 drops to spine 2x daily.

Probiotic Complex
Take 2 capsules in the morning on an empty stomach.

Grounding Blend
Carry throughout the day and apply to temples as needed.

Additional Support
• Siberian Fir

Blood Pressure (high)

Description
Regulates blood pressure by dilation of blood vessels and reducing the viscosity of the blood.

Suggested Duration
6-12 months

Cypress, Marjoram, Ylang Ylang, Lemon
Apply a drop of each over the chest and bottom of feet 2x daily.

Marjoram, Ylang Ylang, Lemon, Yarrow
Take 2 drops each in a capsule 2x daily.

Additional Support
• Clary Sage
• Lavender
• Cellular Complex

Bronchitis/ Pneumonia

Description
Increases immune response to address possible infections and open the airways for symptomatic relief.

Suggested Duration
1-2 weeks

Cardamom, Black Pepper, Rosemary, Lime
Apply drop of each to chest and bottoms of feet 3-5x daily.

Respiratory Blend
Diffuse several drops; inhale 2 drops from cupped hands as needed.

Protective Blend Softgels +
Take 2 softgels 2x daily until symptoms subside.

Additional Support
• Arborvitae
• Oregano

Cancer

Description
Increases the immune response and slows the growth of abnormal cell proliferation.

Suggested Duration
1-3 years

Cellular Complex
Apply 2-4 drops to back of neck, spine, and bottoms of feet 4x daily.

Frankincense, Sandalwood, Turmeric, Lemongrass
Take a drop of each in a capsule 4x daily.

Detoxification Blend
Apply 2 drops diluted to sides of neck 3x daily.

Probiotic Complex
Take 2 capsules in the morning on an empty stomach.

Additional Support
• Detoxification Blend Softgels
• Detox Herbal Complex

Candida (Yeast)

Description
Combats fungus overgrowth in gut, restores healthy flora.

Suggested Duration
2-3 months

Melaleuca, Lavender, Thyme, Clove
Dilute with a carrier oil and apply a drop of each to vaginal area 6x daily. (Follow the same protocol if infection is on the face or body.)

Probiotic Complex
Take 2 capsules in the morning and evening on an empty stomach.

Digestive Blend
2 softgels 2x daily after food.

Additional Support
• Arborvitae
• Yarrow
• Green Mandarin

Canker Sores

Description
Decreases the expression of the virus and maintains a preventative regimen.

Suggested Duration
2-4 weeks

Melaleuca, Oregano, Clove
Dilute a drop each with FCO and apply directly to canker sore. Hold in mouth for 3 minutes. Apply 6x daily.

Combine 3 drops each to 20 drops of carrier oil and swish for 2 minutes daily for ongoing prevention.

Probiotic Complex
Take 2 capsules in the morning and evening on an empty stomach.

Protective Blend Softgels +
Take 2 softgels 2x daily.

Carpet Deodorizer

Eliminates carpet odors from food and pets.

As needed

Cleansing Blend, Lemon, Lime, Melaleuca
Combine 5 drops each with 1 cup baking soda. Rub evenly throughout carpet, and let sit for 12-24 hours before vacuuming.

• Grapefruit
• Bergamot
• Douglas Fir

Celiac's

Promotes nutrient absorption, calms digestive system.

Ongoing

Digestive Enzymes
Take 2-3 capsules with meals.

Probiotic Complex
Take 2 capsules morning and evening on an empty stomach.

Digestive Blend
Rub on outside of stomach at onset of pain.

Metabolic Blend Softgels
Take 1-2 softgels 2-3x daily.

• Cinnamon
• Grapefruit
• Frankincense

Cholesterol (high)

Reduces the amount of cholesterol in the blood to prevent the formation of clots that may lead to heart conditions.

6-12 months

Yarrow, Rosemary, Frankincense
Take 2 drops each in a capsule 2x daily.

Vitality Trio
Take 2 of each bottle 2x daily.

Cellular Complex
Apply 2-4 drops to bottoms of feet 2x daily.

Probiotic Complex
Take 2 capsules morning and evening on an empty stomach.

• Digestive Blend Softgels
• Turmeric

Protocols

Cold Sores

Description
Combats viral infection, and promotes skin healing and pain relief.

Suggested Duration
As needed

Melaleuca & Melissa
Apply a drop of each diluted several times a day to combat the virus.

Helichrysum
Apply a drop diluted at night to help tissue heal.

Probiotic Complex
Take 2 capsules in the morning on an empty stomach.

Additional Support
• Arborvitae
• Black Pepper
• Protective Blend
• Frankincense

Colds

Description
Provides antiviral and respiratory support.

Suggested Duration
5-10 days

Protective Blend Softgels +
Take 2 softgels 3x daily.

Protective Blend, Black Pepper, Melaleuca
Rub 2 drops each on bottoms of feet 3x daily.

Respiratory Blend
Rub onto chest and diffuse as needed.

Vitality Supplement Trio
Take 2 of each bottle 2x daily.

Additional Support
• Rosemary
• Cardamom
• Lime
• Litsea
• Energy & Stamina Complex

Cough

Description
Increases immune response to address possible infections; opens the airways for symptomatic relief.

Suggested Duration
1-2 weeks

Cardamom & Lime
Gargle a drop each with water for 30 seconds, then swallow 3x daily.

Respiratory Blend, Rosemary, Black Pepper
Apply 2 drops each to chest and bottoms of feet 2x daily. Also diffuse several drops throughout the day.

Protective Blend Softgels +
Take 2 softgels 2x daily until symptoms subside.

Additional Support
• Oregano
• Melissa
• Arborvitae

Protocols

Crohn's

Reduces inflammation and swelling in the bowels.

6 months

GI Cleansing Complex
Take 1 softgel 1-2x daily for 2 weeks.

Peppermint, Basil, Frankincense
Take 1-2 drops each in capsule daily for 2 weeks after GI Cleansing Complex.

Probiotic Complex
Take 1 capsule w/each meal.

Digestive Blend
Take 1 softgel to ease discomfort 3-5x daily.

Additional Support
• Vitality Supplement Trio
• Ginger
• Marjoram

Deodorant (body)

Helps manage bacteria and odor-causing toxicity.

4 weeks, then as needed

Cilantro
Take 2 drops in a capsule daily.

Detoxification Softgels
Take 1 softgel 2x daily.

Cleansing Blend
Use diluted with carrier oil under arms after showering.

Additional Support
• Joyful Blend
• Melaleuca
• Arborvitae
• Petitgrain

Depression

Increases mood by stimulation through senses.

3 months, then as needed

Bergamot, Melissa, Frankincense
Apply a drop of each to back of neck, spine and bottoms of feet 3x daily.

Joyful Blend
Diffuse several drops daily and inhale from cupped hands as needed.

Probiotic Complex
Take 2 capsules in the morning on an empty stomach.

Vitality Supplement Trio
Take 2 of each bottle 2x daily.

Additional Support
• Uplifting Blend
• Enlightening Blend

Detox (full body)

Description
Helps the body eliminate toxicity and free up filtering organs.

Suggested Duration
4 weeks

GI Cleansing Complex
Take 1 softgel w/each meal for 10 days (start with 1 a day, and work up to 3).

Detoxification Softgels
Take 1 softgel w/each meal.

Detox Herbal Complex
Take 1 capsule 2x daily.

Probiotic Complex
Take 1 capsule w/each meal during last 10 days.

Vitality Supplement Trio
Take 2 of each bottle 2x daily.

Additional Support
• Lemon (in water)

Diabetes (type 1)

Description
Stimulates cellular maintenance, helps balance blood sugar.

Suggested Duration
3-6 months, then as needed

Vitality Supplement Trio
Take 2 of each bottle 2x daily.

Rosemary, Cypress, Cassia
Take 1 drop each in capsule daily. Also rub diluted onto pancreas reflex points.

Geranium & Rosemary
Add 3 drops of each to a hot bath.

Additional Support
• Cellular Complex Blend
• Coriander
• Juniper Berry
• Bergamot

Diabetes (type 2)

Description
Helps balance blood sugar, supports pancreas.

Suggested Duration
3-6 months, then as needed

Coriander, Cinnamon, Juniper Berry
Take 1-2 drops each in capsule daily.

Cellular Vitality Complex
Take 2 of each bottle 2x daily.

Detoxification Blend
Rub 2 drops onto pancreas reflex point or over pancreas daily.

Additional Support
• Cassia
• Metabolic Blend

Digestive Issues

Relieves inflammation, gas, and discomfort in digestive system.

4 weeks, then as needed

Digestive Blend
Drink 1-2 drops with water, or rub over stomach to ease discomfort.

Digestive Enzymes
Take 1 capsule w/each meal.

Probiotic Complex
Take 2 capsules in the morning on an empty stomach.

Frankincense & Cardamom
Rub a drop of each onto stomach reflex points in the morning.

Additional Support
• Ginger
• Fennel
• Yarrow

Eczema/Dermatitis

Description
Reduces the infection, increases moisture, and promotes new skin cell growth.

Suggested Duration
3 months, then as needed

Arborvitae, Melaleuca, Frankincense
Combine 1-2 drops each with FCO and apply to the affected area 5x daily.

Apply a warm towel compress over the area after oils are applied in the evening.

Protective Blend Softgels +
Take 2 softgels 3x daily with food

Probiotic Complex
Take 2 capsules in the morning on an empty stomach.

Additional Support
• Myrrh
• Hawaiian Sandalwood

Fatigue (low energy)

Description
Increases energy by stimulation of the sympathetic nervous system, eliminating toxins, and inducing cellular pruning and regeneration.

Suggested Duration
6 months, then as needed

Peppermint, Bergamot, Lemongrass
Apply a drop of each to back of neck, spine and bottom of feet 3x daily.

Energy & Stamina Complex
Take 2 capsules 2x daily.

Probiotic Complex
Take 2 capsules in the morning on an empty stomach.

Omega Complex
Take 2 capsules 2x daily.

Additional Support
• Vitality Supplement Trio
• Peppermint

Protocols

Fibromyalgia

Decreases inflammation, promotes healthy cellular function.

1-3 years

Frankincense, Yarrow, Copaiba, Turmeric
Apply a drop of each to back of neck and bottoms of feet 2x daily.

Cellular Complex
Apply 2-4 drops to spine 2x daily. Also take 2 softgels 2x daily.

Soothing Blend
Massage lotion into inflamed areas 3x daily or as needed.

Probiotic Complex
Take 2 capsules in the morning on an empty stomach.

Melissa
Use 1 drop under tongue daily.

• Vitality Supplement Trio

Flu Bomb

Combats viruses, boosts immune system, supports respiratory system.

5-10 days

Protective Blend, Melaleuca, Black Pepper
Rub 2 drops each on bottoms of feet 3x daily.

Protective Blend Softgels +
Take 2 softgels 3x daily.

Digestive Blend
Drink 1-3 drops in water, or rub over stomach to ease nausea & vomiting.

Respiratory Blend
Diffuse 8-10 drops. Sit/sleep near the diffuser. Also rub 2 drops over chest as needed.

• Melissa
• GI Cleansing Complex

Heartburn

Balances stomach acid, eases pain of indigestion.

As needed

Digestive Blend
Drink 1-2 drops in water.

Digestive Enzymes
Take 1-3 capsules with each meal.

Cardamom
Rub 1-2 drops over stomach.

• Ginger
• Fennel
• Coriander

Protocols

Immune Boost

Provides bacteria and virus-fighting agents, boosts immune system.

4 weeks

Protective Blend, Black Pepper, Melaleuca
Rub 2-4 drops each on bottoms of feet daily.

Probiotic Complex
Take 2 capsules in the morning on an empty stomach.

Vitality Supplement Trio
Take 2 of each bottle 2x daily.

• Frankincense
• Melissa
• Thyme

Infertility

Supports the reproductive system and proper hormone production.

2-6 months

Full Body Detox
Follow instructions for Detox (full body).

Vitality Supplement Trio
Take 2 of each bottle 2x daily.

Clary Sage
Apply to reproductive reflex points 2x daily.

Yarrow
Take 2 drops under tongue 2x daily.

• Oil Touch Technique (receive weekly)
• Detoxification Blend

Irritable Bowels (IBS)

Relieves symptoms of gas, bloating, constipation, diarrhea, and belching.

3-6 months

Digestive Blend
Take 1 softgel after 2 meals.

Cardamom & Turmeric
Drink a drop each in water to soothe discomfort as needed.

Probiotic Complex
Take 2 capsules in the morning and evening on an empty stomach.

Omega Complex
2 softgels 2x daily.

Lavender, Melaleuca, Frankincense, Digestive Blend
Apply a drop of each diluted over stomach 2x daily.

• Fennel
• Coriander

Protocols

Libido (sex drive)

Inspires an uninhibited sex drive.

2 weeks, then as needed

Inspiring Blend
Use a few drops diluted in massage, and diffuse several drops to inspire intimacy.

Ylang Ylang
Rub 1-2 drops on pulse points.

Clary Sage
Take 1-2 drops in capsule daily.

· Vitality Supplement Trio
· Energy & Stamina Complex
· Women's Perfume Blend

Lupus

Induces the parasympathetic nervous system, eliminates antigens and latent infections, and reduces the immune response.

1-3 years

Frankincense, Yarrow, Copaiba, Turmeric
Apply a drop of each to back of neck and bottoms of feet 2x daily.

Cellular Complex
Apply 2-4 drops to spine 2x daily. Also take 2 softgels 2x daily.

Soothing Blend
Massage lotion into inflamed areas 3x daily or as needed.

Probiotic Complex
Take 2 capsules in the morning on an empty stomach.

· Vitality Supplement Trio

Lyme Disease

Induces the parasympathetic nervous system, eliminates antigens and latent infections, and reduces the immune response.

1-3 years

Cellular Complex
Apply 2-4 drops to spine, back of neck, and bottoms of feet 3x daily.

Cinnamon, Sandalwood, Turmeric, Clary Sage
Take a drop of each in a capsule 2x daily.

Detoxification Blend
Apply 2 drops to sides of neck 2x daily.

Probiotic Complex
Take 2 capsules in the morning on an empty stomach.

Copaiba Softgels
Take 1 softgel 3x daily.

· Vitality Supplement Trio
· Yarrow

Menopause

Aids in hormone and mood balance, calms hot flashes.

4 months, then as needed

Women's Monthly Blend
Rub onto pulse points twice daily (avoid sun exposure for 12 hours after application).

Phytoestrogen Complex
Take 1 capsule 3x daily.

Peppermint
Apply a drop to back of neck to ease hot flashes.

• Vitality Supplement Trio
• Ylang Ylang
• Geranium

Menstruation

Balances mood and hormones during menstruation.

2 weeks as needed

Women's Monthly Blend
Rub onto pulse points and over ovaries (avoid sun exposure for 12 hours after application).

Balance
Rub behind ears to balance mood.

Phytoestrogen
Take 1 capsule 3x daily.

• Clary Sage
• Restful Blend
• Tension Blend

Mononucleosis

Provides antiviral support.

8-16 weeks

Thyme, Oregano, Protective Blend
Take 1-2 drops each in a capsule 3x daily.

Frankincense, Black Pepper
Rub 2 drops each to bottoms of feet.

Energy & Stamina Complex
Take 1-2 capsules twice daily.

• Vitality Supplement Trio
• Melissa
• Cassia

Protocols

Muscle Aches

Description
Reduces inflammation, spasms, and pain in muscles.

Suggested Duration
2 weeks, then as needed

Massage Blend
Massage 2-4 drops into aching muscles 3x daily.

Polyphenol Complex
Take 1 capsule 3x daily.

Frankincense, Lemon
Take 1-2 drops each in capsule 2x daily.

Magnolia
Apply to affected muscles as needed throughout the day.

Additional Support
• Soothing Blend
• Cypress
• Douglas Fir
• Black Pepper

Pregnancy (postnatal)

Description
Promotes pain relief, tissue healing, and emotional support after giving birth.

Suggested Duration
4-8 weeks

Helichrysum, Frankincense, Lavender
Apply 2 drops each diluted to areas with tearing 3x daily.

Ylang Ylang
Diffuse for mood balancing.

Phytoestrogen
Take 1 capsule 3x daily.

Helichrysum, Myrrh, Lavender
Massage 2 drops each diluted into stretch mark areas.

Additional Support
• Geranium
• Vitality Supplement Trio

Pregnancy (prenatal)

Description
Relieves pregnancy sickness, provides vital nutrients, and provides emotional support.

Suggested Duration
9 months

Digestive Blend
Drink 2 drops or rub 2 drops over stomach to ease nausea.

Digestive Enzymes
Take 1-3 w/each meal.

Vitality Supplement Trio
Take 2 of each bottle 2x daily.

Bone Nutrient Complex
Take 1 capsule 3x daily.

Joyful Blend
Diffuse or wear daily.

Additional Support
• Ginger
• Grounding Blend
• Metabolic Blend

Psoriasis

Relieves itchy, swollen skin, and promotes proper immune system function.

4-8 weeks

Helichrysum, Frankincense, Melaleuca, Lavender
Combine 10 drops each with carrier oil in roller bottle. Apply 3x daily.

Probiotic Complex
Take 2 capsules in the morning on an empty stomach.

Digestive Enzymes
Take 1-3 w/each meal.

Cellular Complex Blend
Take 1-2 softgels 3x daily.

Additional Support
• Copaiba
• Anti-Aging Blend
• Cedarwood

Shingles

Description
Decreases the expression of the viral infection, alleviates pain, and maintains a preventative regiment.

Suggested Duration
1 week to 3 months

Cardamom, Melissa, Lemon Myrtle, Melaleuca
Apply a drop of each with carrier oil to blisters 6x daily.

Probiotic Complex
Take 2 capsules morning and evening on an empty stomach.

Protective Blend
Take 2 capsules 2x daily after food.

Omega Complex
Take 2 softgels 2x daily.

Additional Support
• Seasonal Blend Softgels
• Vitality Supplement Trio

Sinusitis

Description
Clears the bacterial infections and assists in the remediation of the symptoms.

Suggested Duration
1-4 weeks

Cardamom, Rosemary, Arborvitae, Melissa
Apply a drop of each with carrier oil over the maxillary sinus region 6x daily.

Probiotic Complex
Take 2 capsules morning and evening on an empty stomach.

Protective Blend
Take 2 capsules 2x daily after food.

Omega Complex
Take 2 softgels 2x daily.

Additional Support
• Myrrh
• Oregano

Protocols

Sleep (Insomnia)

Description
Induces a calming state that allows one to fall and stay asleep.

Suggested Duration
3 months, then as needed

Restful Blend Complex
Take 2 softgels 30 minutes before bed.

Restful Blend
Apply 2 drops to temples and bottoms of feet. Diffuse several drops near bedside.

Vetiver & Wild Orange
Take a drop of each under the tongue before bed.

Probiotic Complex
Take 2 capsules in the morning on an empty stomach.

Additional Support
- Frankincense
- Sandalwood
- Wild Orange

Sleep Apnea

Description
Promotes open airways and more meaningful sleep.

Suggested Duration
Ongoing

Respiratory Blend
Diffuse 5-10 drops next to bedside at night. Also apply to sinus reflex points.

Protective Blend
Gargle 2 drops with water for 30 seconds, then swallow.

Restful Complex
Take 2 softgels 30 minutes before bed.

Additional Support
- Peppermint
- Rosemary
- Wintergreen

Smoking

Description
Helps curb cravings and smoking addiction, aids in detox.

Suggested Duration
6-12 weeks

Grapefruit
Drink 1-3 drops in water throughout the day.

Protective Blend
Swish 2 drops with water when cravings arise, especially after eating.

Black Pepper
Apply 1 drop to big toes 2x daily. Also inhale or diffuse throughout the day.

Detoxification Blend
Apply 2-4 drops to bottoms of feet 30 minutes before showering.

Additional Support
- Detox Herbal Complex

Snoring

Description
Promotes open airways during sleep.

Suggested Duration
Ongoing

Respiratory Blend
Diffuse 5-10 drops near bedside at night. Also apply to chest, throat, and lung reflex points.

Protective Blend
Gargle 2 drops with water for 30 seconds, then swallow.

Lemon
Drink 1-3 drops in water before bed.

Additional Support
- Eucalyptus
- Rosemary
- Peppermint

Sore Throat

Description
Relieves pain and soreness in throat, provides antiviral and antibacterial support.

Suggested Duration
5-10 days

Lemon 10, Protective Blend 8, Helichrysum 2
Combine in small glass spray bottle with carrier oil. Apply as needed.

Lavender, Arborvitae
Massage 1-2 drops with carrier oil to outside of throat.

Additional Support
- Melissa
- Black Pepper
- Petitgrain

Stress

Description
Increases a general calming state due to the interaction of oils with neurotransmitters.

Suggested Duration
4-8 weeks, then as needed

Grounding Blend
Apply 1-2 drops to back of ears, temples, and wrists often as needed.

Grapefruit, Tangerine, or Wild Orange
Diffuse several drops daily.

Probiotic Complex
Take 2 capsules in the morning on an empty stomach.

Restful Blend
Apply 2-4 drops to temples and bottoms of feet at bedtime. Diffuse several drops.

Additional Support
- Rose

Protocols

179

Sunburn

Relieves discomfort from sunburn, promotes healing.

Suggested Duration
3-7 days

Lavender, Yarrow, Helichrysum
Apply 2-4 drops with carrier oil or aloe to sunburnt skin 3-5x daily.

Peppermint
Add 5 drops to small glass spray bottle with water. Spritz to cool skin.

Additional Support
- Cedarwood
- Copaiba
- Roman Chamomile

Thrush

Description
Provides anti-fungal support, eases oral discomfort.

Suggested Duration
1-3 weeks

Lemon, Melaleuca, Children's Omega-3
Combine 2 drops of each essential oil with 1 Tbs of omegas. Apply with clean finger to child's gums and tongue 2-3x daily.

Melaleuca & Lavender
Massage a drop into bottoms of child's feet 1x daily.

Additional Support
- Geranium
- Helichrysum

Thyroid: Hyper (Grave's)

Description
Assists with regulating the metabolism, detoxifying the body, and restoring balance.

Suggested Duration
1-3 years

Vetiver, Siberian Fir, Turmeric, Myrrh
Apply a drop of each to back of neck, spine, and throat 3x daily.

Probiotic Complex
Take 2 capsules in the morning on an empty stomach.

Grounding Blend
Apply 2-4 drops to bottoms of feet morning and night.

Detoxification Blend
Take 2 softgels 2x daily.

Additional Support
- Sandalwood
- Detox Herbal Complex

Thyroid: Hypo (Hashimoto's)

Assists with regulating the metabolism, detoxifying the body, and restoring balance.

1-3 years

Myrrh, Turmeric, Clove, Lemongrass, Copaiba
Apply a drop of each to back of neck, spine, and throat 3x daily.

Probiotic Complex
Take 2 capsules in the morning on an empty stomach.

Energy & Stamina Complex
Take 2 capsules 2x daily.

Detoxification Blend
Take 2 softgels 2x daily.

Cellular Complex Softgels
Take 2 softgels 2x daily.

• Rosemary

Weight loss

Assists with burning glucose and glycogen supplies at a faster rate in order to access the ketotic fat burning state.

3-6 months

Metabolic Blend
Apply 10-15 drops with carrier oil to abdomen and fatty areas at night.

Also drink 3-5 drops in water throughout the day.

Cellular Complex
Apply 2-4 drops of oil to lower abdomen 2x daily. Take 2 softgels 2x daily.

Detoxification Blend Softgels
Take 2 softgels 2x daily.

• Bergamot
• Coriander
• Fennel

Workout

Provides pre- and post-workout support, increases energy, supports muscle tone.

Ongoing

Massage Blend
Apply 1-3 drops to muscles to stimulate circulation before workout.

Respiratory Blend
Apply 2-4 drops to chest to open airways.

Energy & Stamina Complex
Take 2 capsules before workout, and 2 with dinner.

Soothing Blend
Apply in lotion to muscles and joints after workout. Add Marjoram if injured.

• Lemongrass
• Vitality Supplement Trio

Bibliography

Aromatic Science. AromaticScience, LLC. Web. July, 2017. <www.aromaticscience.com>

AromaTools. Modern Essentials: a Contemporary Guide to the Therapeutic Use of Essential Oils. Aroma-Tools, 2018.

Enlighten Alternative Healing. Emotions and Essential Oils: A Modern Resource for Healing: Emotional Reference Guide. 4th ed., Enlighten Alternative Healing, 2017.

Harding, Jennie: The Essential Oils Handbook. Duncan Baird Publishers Ltd, 2008.

Lawless, Julia: The Encyclopedia of Essential Oils: The Complete Guide to the Use of Aromatic Oils In Aromatherapy, Herbalism, Health, and Well Being. Conari Press, 2013.

Schiller, Carol & Schiller, David: The Aromatherapy Encyclopedia: A Concise Guide to Over 395 Plant Oils. Basic Health Publications Inc, 2008.

Schnaubelt, Kurt. The Healing Intelligence of Essential Oils: the Science of Advanced Aromatherapy. Healing Arts Press, 2011.

Tisserand, Robert, et al. Essential Oil Safety: A Guide for Health Care Professionals. 2nd ed., Churchill Livingstone/Elsevier, 2014.

Total Wellness Publishing. The Essential Life: A Simple Guide to Living the Wellness Lifestyle. Total Wellness Publishing, 2017.

Worwood, Valerie Ann. The Complete Book of Essential Oils and Aromatherapy, Revised and Expanded: Over 800 Natural, Nontoxic, and Fragrant Recipes to Create Health, Beauty, And Safe Home and Work Environments. New World Library, 2016.

Oil Magic Publishing would also like to thank the up-and-coming photographers on Unsplash, whose work can be found on some of the pages of this book. Visit www.oilmagicbook.com to see full credits.

Section 8

Protocols
for Sharing

ADD/ADHD

Description
Increases focus and concentration, supports healthy hormones and brain chemistry.

Suggested Duration
Ongoing

Vitality Supplement Trio
Take 2 of each bottle 2x/day.

Focus Blend
Carry in your pocket, and roll a small amount on back of neck as needed for focus.

Grounding Blend
Apply 2 drops to bottoms of feet each morning.

Probiotic Complex
Take 1 with each meal.

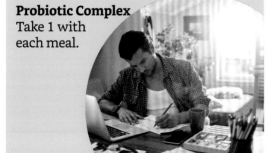

ADD/ADHD

Description
Increases focus and concentration, supports healthy hormones and brain chemistry.

Suggested Duration
Ongoing

Vitality Supplement Trio
Take 2 of each bottle 2x/day.

Focus Blend
Carry in your pocket, and roll a small amount on back of neck as needed for focus.

Grounding Blend
Apply 2 drops to bottoms of feet each morning.

Probiotic Complex
Take 1 with each meal.

"Health is the greatest gift, content-
ment is the greatest wealth, faithful-
ness the best relationship."

–Buddha

This protocol is
brought to you by the book
Essential Oil Magic

"A calm mind brings inner strength
and self-confidence."

–Dalai Lama

This protocol is
brought to you by the book
Essential Oil Magic

Allergies

Description
Reduces histamine response, boosts immune response.

Suggested Duration
4-8 weeks to begin, then as needed

Lemon, Lavender, Peppermint
Put 1 drop each under tongue. Drink water after 30 seconds.

Respiratory Blend
Inhale from cupped hands when experiencing attack.

Probiotic Complex
Take 1 capsule 3x/day.

Protective Blend
Gargle 2 drops with water nightly, then swallow.

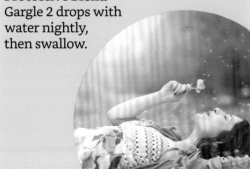

Allergies

Description
Reduces histamine response, boosts immune response.

Suggested Duration
4-8 weeks to begin, then as needed

Lemon, Lavender, Peppermint
Put 1 drop each under tongue. Drink water after 30 seconds.

Respiratory Blend
Inhale from cupped hands when experiencing attack.

Probiotic Complex
Take 1 capsule 3x/day.

Protective Blend
Gargle 2 drops with water nightly, then swallow.

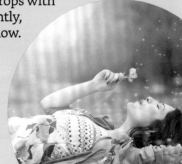

"In three words I can sum up every-
thing I've learned about life: It goes
on."

-Robert Frost

This protocol is
brought to you by the book
Essential Oil Magic

"As for butter versus margarine, I
trust cows more than chemists."

-Joan Gussow

This protocol is
brought to you by the book
Essential Oil Magic

Anxiety & Stress

Description
Reduces stress levels, promotes sense of calm, security, and focus.

Suggested Duration
3-6 months, then as needed

Grounding Blend
Apply 2 drops to bottoms of feet in mornings. Rub a drop behind ears when anxious.

Frankincense
Put a drop under tongue. Drink water after 30 seconds.

Reassuring Blend
Apply to pulse points and temples as needed.

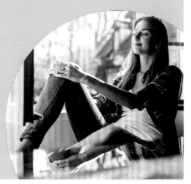

Anxiety & Stress

Description
Reduces stress levels, promotes sense of calm, security, and focus.

Suggested Duration
3-6 months, then as needed

Grounding Blend
Apply 2 drops to bottoms of feet in mornings. Rub a drop behind ears when anxious.

Frankincense
Put a drop under tongue. Drink water after 30 seconds.

Reassuring Blend
Apply to pulse points and temples as needed.

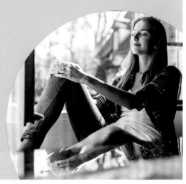

"We make a living by what we get. We make a life by what we give."

-Winston Churchill

This protocol is
brought to you by the book

Essential Oil Magic

"It's not who you are that holds you back, it's who you think you're not."

-Denis Waitley

This protocol is
brought to you by the book

Essential Oil Magic

Back, Neck, & Shoulder Pain

Reduces pain and inflammation, promotes mobility.

4 weeks, then as needed

Soothing Blend
Massage in lotion into affected areas often as needed.

Polyphenol Complex
Take 1 capsule 3x/day.

Marjoram
Massage 1-2 drops into any injured muscles.

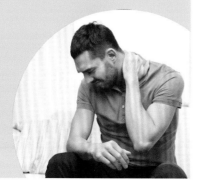

Back, Neck, & Shoulder Pain

Description
Reduces pain and inflammation, promotes mobility.

Suggested Duration
4 weeks, then as needed

Soothing Blend
Massage in lotion into affected areas often as needed.

Polyphenol Complex
Take 1 capsule 3x/day.

Marjoram
Massage 1-2 drops into any injured muscles.

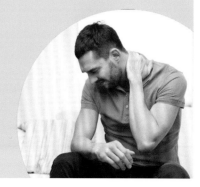

"Nothing is impossible. The word itself says *I'm possible*."

This protocol is
brought to you by the book

"If you obey all the rules, you miss all the fun."

This protocol is
brought to you by the book

Colds

Description
Provides antiviral and respiratory support.

Suggested Duration
5-10 days

Protective Blend
Drink 1-3 drops with water 3x/day.

Protective Blend, Black Pepper, Melaleuca
Rub 1-2 drops each on bottoms of feet 3x/day.

Respiratory Blend
Rub onto chest and diffuse as needed.

Vitality Supplement Trio
Take 2 of each bottle 2x/day.

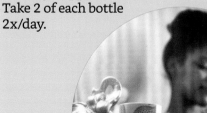

Colds

Description
Provides antiviral and respiratory support.

Suggested Duration
5-10 days

Protective Blend
Drink 1-3 drops with water 3x/day.

Protective Blend, Black Pepper, Melaleuca
Rub 1-2 drops each on bottoms of feet 3x/day.

Respiratory Blend
Rub onto chest and diffuse as needed.

Vitality Supplement Trio
Take 2 of each bottle 2x/day.

"Motivation will always beat mere talent."

This protocol is
brought to you by the book

"Don't suffer from insanity, enjoy every minute of it."

This protocol is
brought to you by the book

Depression

Description
Improves brain chemistry, supports healthy hormone production.

Suggested Duration
3-6 months, then as needed

Joyful Blend
Carry with you, and inhale from cupped hands often as needed for mood support.

Frankincense or Melissa
Put a drop under the tongue 1-3x/day.

Vitality Supplement Trio
Take 2 of each bottle 2x/day.

Also consider Essential Oils + Omegas and the Probiotic Complex.

Depression

Description
Improves brain chemistry, supports healthy hormone production.

Suggested Duration
3-6 months, then as needed

Joyful Blend
Carry with you, and inhale from cupped hands often as needed for mood support.

Frankincense or Melissa
Put a drop under the tongue 1-3x/day.

Vitality Supplement Trio
Take 2 of each bottle 2x/day.

Also consider Essential Oils + Omegas and the Probiotic Complex.

"Your imagination is your preview to
life's coming attractions."

-Albert Einstein

This protocol is
brought to you by the book
Essential Oil Magic

"Success is getting what you want.
Happiness is wanting what you get."

-Dale Carnegie

This protocol is
brought to you by the book
Essential Oil Magic

Digestive Issues

Description
Relieves inflammation, gas, and discomfort in digestive system.

Suggested Duration
2-4 weeks, then as needed

Digestive Blend
Drink 1-2 drops with water, or rub over stomach to ease discomfort.

Digestive Enzymes
Take 1 capsule w/each meal.

Probiotic Complex
Take 1 capsule w/each meal.

Frankincense & Cardamom
Rub a drop of each onto stomach reflex points in the morning.

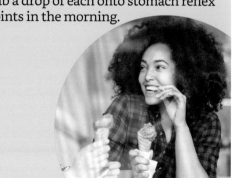

"People often say that motivation doesn't last. Well, neither does bathing; that's why we recommend it daily."

-Zig Ziglar

This protocol is
brought to you by the book
Essential Oil Magic

"A fit, healthy body -- That is the best fashion statement."

-Jess C. Scott

This protocol is
brought to you by the book
Essential Oil Magic

Fatigue

Description
Supports adrenals, micro-circulation, and alertness.

Suggested Duration
4 weeks, then as needed

Peppermint & Rosemary
Apply 2 drops to bottoms of feet daily. Inhale from cupped hands as needed.

Lemon or Grapefruit
Use 1-3 drops in water 3x/day.

Vitality Supplement Trio
Take 2 of each bottle 2x/day.

Energy & Stamina Complex
Take 2 capsules 2x/day.

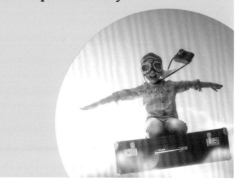

Fatigue

Description
Supports adrenals, micro-circulation, and alertness.

Suggested Duration
4 weeks, then as needed

Peppermint & Rosemary
Apply 2 drops to bottoms of feet daily. Inhale from cupped hands as needed.

Lemon or Grapefruit
Use 1-3 drops in water 3x/day.

Vitality Supplement Trio
Take 2 of each bottle 2x/day.

Energy & Stamina Complex
Take 2 capsules 2x/day.

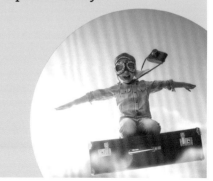

"You live only once, but if you do it right, once is enough."

—Mae West

This protocol is
brought to you by the book
Essential Oil Magic

"A healthy attitude is contagious, but don't wait to catch it from others; be a carrier."

—Tom Stoppard

This protocol is
brought to you by the book
Essential Oil Magic

Flu Bomb

Description
Combats viruses, boosts immune system, supports respiratory system.

Suggested Duration
5-10 days

Oregano, Melaleuca, Protective Blend, Lemon
Take 1-2 drops of each in a capsule 3x/day.

Digestive Blend
Drink 1-3 drops in water, or rub over stomach to ease nausea & vomiting.

Respiratory Blend
Diffuse 8-10 drops. Sit/sleep near the diffuser.

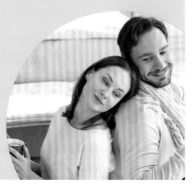

Flu Bomb

Description
Combats viruses, boosts immune system, supports respiratory system.

Suggested Duration
5-10 days

Oregano, Melaleuca, Protective Blend, Lemon
Take 1-2 drops of each in a capsule 3x/day.

Digestive Blend
Drink 1-3 drops in water, or rub over stomach to ease nausea & vomiting.

Respiratory Blend
Diffuse 8-10 drops. Sit/sleep near the diffuser.

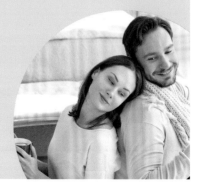

"If you're happy, if you're feeling good, then nothing else matters."

-Robin Wright

This protocol is
brought to you by the book
Essential Oil Magic

"The produce manager is more important to my children's health than the pediatrician."

-Meryl Streep

This protocol is
brought to you by the book
Essential Oil Magic